THE

Miracle Foods

COOKBOOK

ॐ ॐ ॐ

Easy, Low-Cost Recipes and Menus with Antioxidant-Rich Vegetables and Fruits that Help you Lose Weight, Fight Disease, and Slow the Aging Process.

M.J. Smith, R.D.

CHRONIMED
PUBLISHING

The Miracle Foods Cookbook: *Easy, low-cost recipes and menus with antioxidant-rich vegetables and fruits that help you lose weight, fight disease, and slow the aging process.* ©1995 by M.J. Smith, R.D.

Library of Congress Cataloging-in-Publication Data

Smith, M.J. (Margaret Jane), 1955-
The Miracle Foods Cookbook: Easy, low-cost recipes and menus with antioxidant-rich vegetables and fruits that help you lose weight, fight disease, and slow the aging process / M.J. Smith, R.D.

P.   cm.
Includes index
ISBN 1-56561-056-3; $12.95
1. Low-fat diet—Recipes.

I. Title.
XX000.0.X00 1995
000.0'000—dc00 00 00000
                CIP

Edited by: Donna Hoel
Cover Design: Terry Dugan Design
Text Design: Liana Viaciulis Raudys
Art/Production Manager: Claire Lewis
Production Artist: Janet Hogge
Printed in the United States of America

Published by
CHRONIMED Publishing, Inc.
P.O. Box 47945
Minneapolis, MN 55447-9727

DEDICATION

There are many fruits on the tree of life, but none so sweet as friendship. This book is dedicated to the miracle of friendship and my friend, Mary Kay Long Finch.

Mary was a continuing source of encouragement and inspiration when I complained about cookbook deadlines or computer foul ups. She loved fruits and vegetables. For three years through humid Iowa summers and below-zero winters, we would meet each other at 6:15 a.m. on Acre Street and take our 30-minute walk. She always greeted me with "grapefruit breath" because that was her wake-up food. As a pre-school teacher, she would lunch quickly and quietly on an apple or a banana between classes. We shared a love of coleslaw and enjoyed many lunches out, with orders of CLTs (grilled chicken, lettuce and tomato sandwiches) and slaw.

Mary died during the last month of my writing this book. She has enriched my life with memories and wisdom as few friends do, and for that reason I am recording them in this dedication.

WISDOM OF MARY KAY

I don't care who started this fight, I want to know who is ending it.

I have friends I haven't even met yet.

Things always seem to work out for me.

Let go and let God.

No duds allowed at this party!

Do it, do it right, and do it right now.

ACKNOWLEDGMENTS

Special thanks to:

Ms. Kate Merrick who analyzed recipes for nutrient value.

Ms. Alice Jane Walter for editorial comment.

Ms. Cindy Crow who typed through the night.

To my husband, the gardener, who provided some delicious main ingredients for recipe testing.

ABOUT THE AUTHOR

M. J. Smith is a consultant dietitian and cookbook author from Guttenberg, Iowa. Her previous books include: *All American Low-Fat Meals in Minutes, 60 Days of Low Cost Low-Fat Meals in Minutes, and 366 Low-Fat Brand-Name Recipes in Minutes.*

After fifteen years of helping clients make food choices for better health, she has developed a passion for spreading the news about fruits and vegetables. This book was inspired by her clients who answered "corn, beans, and peas" when asked, "Tell me about the vegetables in your diet."

Ms. Smith is convinced now more than ever that many of the evolving mysteries in nutrition will be answered by fruits and vegetables.

The author is married to Dr. Andy Smith, a family physician, and they have two school-aged children. Her favorite fruits are watermelon and raspberries, and her favorite vegetable is cabbage.

Even if I knew certainly the world would end tomorrow, I would plant an apple tree today.

—Martin Luther

TABLE OF CONTENTS

RECIPES:

Appetizers

Beverages

Soups

Fruit Soups

Fruit Salads

Vegetable Salads

INTRODUCTION

I have become a true believer in the gospel of fruits and vegetables.

In 1993, over one million new cases of cancer were diagnosed and over half a million people died of cancer in the United States.

1. Cancer experts attribute one in three cancer cases to unhealthful dietary patterns.

2. More specifically, they cite diets that are:

   —high in fat,
   —low in fiber, and
   —low in fruits and vegetables.

Excellent studies from many countries using a variety of research methods have linked these diet patterns to cancers of the pharynx, larynx, esophagus, oral cavity, stomach, pancreas, colon, rectum, lung, bladder, endometrium, cervix and ovaries.

As a practicing dietitian, I have cared for retired farmers with colon cancer and leukemia and women in the prime of life with breast cancer. My practice and research have deepened my commitment to the value of fruits and vegetables in our diet. Like the majority of my readers, I recall early preaching from my mother about "cleaning up" my green beans. And now after 15 years of counseling practice and hundreds of diet histories, my appreciation and understanding of her advice have evolved into an all-consuming passion.

I believe our traditional views of the role of vitamins from food have been too limited.

The first wave of nutrition research was the discovery of vitamins and their role in combating deficiencies such as rickets and beriberi. Now a second wave of evidence suggests vitamins from food play a more complex role in ensuring optimal health than was previously appreciated by the scientific community.

It does not matter if the diagnosis is hiatal hernia or diabetes, I always work my own "fruit and vegetable sermon" into a diet consultation. Beyond protection from cancer, fruits and vegetables promote a **day-to-day vitality**, including enhanced immune function, protection from heart disease, and aid with weight control. In this book, these benefits are fully discussed in terms you will understand.

I have enjoyed a twofold challenge educating clients about fruits and vegetables:

• first, convincing them optimal intake extends beyond orange juice, mashed potatoes, corn on the cob, and green beans, and

• second, sharing many little-known tricks for serving something new with ease and good and taste.

This book, based on hands-on experience as well as current research, answers these questions:

• How much fruit juice is considered one serving?

• What are "phytochemicals?"

• How should fruits and vegetables be cleaned to remove pesticide residue?

• What are the best sources of antioxidants?

• How do you grill vegetables?

• Do boxed potato mixes help meet the need for fruits and vegetables?

- What is jicama?

- How can I build on my love of bananas and strawberries? (Find 10 ways to prepare each!)

- What strategy presents the best chance for successful introduction of vegetables to children?

- Are genetically-altered tomatoes safe?

- What nutrients are in lettuce?

If you "love fruits and vegetables" and are currently eating five servings a day, congratulations! Use this book to discover a new recipe for Brussels sprouts and make it for supper tonight.

On the other hand, if the adequacy of your fruit and vegetable intake is one peck short of a bushel, then check out the index for an old favorite—like coleslaw or seven-layer salad or old-fashioned pea salad. The fat has been reduced from traditional versions, and you can start piling up your plate from here.

The purpose of this book is to share my passion that fruits and vegetables are a simple answer to many of the nutrition challenges we face today.

WORKING TOWARD "FIVE A DAY"

In July of 1992, our government's leading health officer introduced an important program called **"Five a Day."** Together with the National Institutes of Health, the National Cancer Institute, and an organization called Produce for Better Health, then Secretary of Health and Human Services Louis Sullivan called on Americans to increase their consumption of fruits and vegetables to five servings a day by the year 2000.

Surveys confirmed Americans currently eat an average of three and a half servings of fruits and vegetables, which is one and a half short of the minimum needed for good health. Interestingly, women eat four servings a day and men three—thus, the three and a half average for the nation. Since 1992, supermarkets, newspapers, and national magazines have publicized this profoundly simple Five-a-Day message. Five-a-Day research studies are going on in homes, schools, work-place cafeterias, and college campuses, and within health and nutrition programs for women and children. We will soon know more about what works best to increase fruit and vegetable consumption.

Most Americans say they like the taste of fruits and vegetables! What are the most popular choices for the three and a half servings? In order of the frequency of consumption, the list looks like this:

1. green salad
2. orange and grapefruit juice
3. fried potatoes, other potatoes
4. string beans, peas, and corn
5. tomatoes
6. bananas
7. apples and applesauce
8. tomato sauce
9. salsa and
10. other fruit juices

A worrisome result of this same survey shows one fourth of Americans eat their vegetables cooked in some type of fat (like French fries), or with some type of fat added in the form of butter, cream, or cheese sauce. This troublesome habit occurs most often among those who eat the least number of servings! Conversely, people who eat the most fruits and vegetables are the least likely to prepare vegetables in fat or to add fats after cooking. Reduced-fat recipes like "Granny's Green Bean and Mushroom Casserole" are included in this book to meet the need of many people who still prefer their vegetables to wear disguises.

Beyond the "Five-a-Day" survey, food and beverage consumption figures support a dietitian's dread: Americans are drinking 10 soft drinks to every glass of fruit juice! In 1990, 42.5 gallons of soft drink were sold for every person in America, up from 35 gallons in 1980. At the same time, orange juice sales were down to 4 gallons per capita from a high of 5.6 gallons in 1986.

But Americans are living longer and say they want to stay healthy. Time is our most precious commodity and cooking from scratch is slowly becoming a lost art. Food Marketing Institute studies show most Americans spend approximately 20 minutes a day preparing their main meal and predict that by the year 2000, this time will be cut in half. Americans now spend about 10 minutes less to prepare their main meal than they did just 10 years ago. It should not surprise us the market for pre-cut fruits and vegetables is growing at an estimated annual rate of 20 percent! I won't argue with the ease of pouring shredded cabbage out of the bag.

Half of Americans believe fruits and vegetables will help prevent cancer and heart disease, and will help them lose or maintain weight. However, the awareness of fruit and vegetable benefits is highest among those who eat the largest quantity.

And what about the next generation? People who have formed the habit of eating fruits and vegetables early in life are more likely to consume more as adults. A recent study of Midwest elementary school children reported kids rate soft drinks (water, sugar, colorings, and flavorings) as their favorite beverage, followed by fruit drinks (water, sugar, and fruit juice), and white and chocolate milk. Favorite after-school snacks are baked goods for 30 percent of youngsters, salted snacks are preferred by 26 percent, candy by 28 percent, ice cream by 11 percent, and fruit by just 10 percent of the kids.

Every parent's challenge is to serve fruits and vegetables appealingly and to encourage the habit of eating fruits and vegetables beginning at an early age to potentially improve the health of our children. It is difficult to know why vegetables are the center of so many dinner-table struggles. Parents who have grown up having vegetables pushed on them pass those same attitudes on. While children innately prefer sweet-tasting foods, they view all new foods equally. The best advice is to present vegetables matter-of-factly to children, enjoy them yourself, and allow the children to experiment on their own. They learn to like them, but it may take 13 trials. If you force the issue, disastrous results occur. The section entitled "Just for Kids" is designed to help you avoid such disasters.

Little Emily's food preferences may be genetically determined. If you dislike broccoli, don't be surprised if your child says "no thank-you." Recent research at the University of Cincinnati found that genetic factors influence preferences for this vegetable, as well as for orange juice. The theory goes that there is an inherited sensitivity to a bitter-tasting chemical found naturally in certain foods. The answer is to just keep serving a variety of fruits and vegetables, because the more kids try them, the more likely they will grow to like them. One rule of thumb I use with my clients is children may have to taste a small amount of a new food up to 12 times before accepting it.

The health benefits for children and adults who eat fruits and vegetables are explained in detail in the next section. If you need no further convincing, skip to the section on serving guidelines and menu suggestions.

BUILDING THE CASE FOR FRUITS AND VEGETABLES—THEIR BENEFITS ARE MIRACULOUS!

When my publisher suggested this fruit and vegetable cookbook be called *The Miracle Foods Cookbook*, my Lutheran hair stood on end. You see, this title goes beyond a dietitian's sense of truth in advertising. But if the title grabbed your attention, then I'm not sorry. A diet rich in vegetables and fruits is not a potion granting long life and eternal well-being. Let us just say that they maximize your potential. After reading this section, you can decide for yourself if the benefits of fruits and vegetables add up to something of a miracle.

THE POWER OF ANTIOXIDANTS IN FRUITS AND VEGETABLES

Nutrition scientists have been working diligently over the last five years to understand dietary antioxidants. These are the vitamins A, C, E, and beta carotene (the beginning form of vitamin A) found in vegetables and fruits, which help fight infection and disease.

A review of some basic chemistry is helpful here. Oxygen is vital for human life. However, oxygen-derived "free radicals" are destructive chemicals and cause damage called oxidation. Everyday examples of oxidation are apples browning when sliced, metal rusting, rubber crumbling, and oils turning rancid. Free-radical damage to cells in our bodies can be caused by internal metabolic processes, such as high blood cholesterol, or by outside sources, such as air pollution, tobacco smoke, car exhaust, and sun exposure. When an excess of free radicals is produced, cells can be damaged, and this damage is a factor in cancer and heart disease. Free-radical damage to cells also directly impacts the natural process we know as aging.

Dietary antioxidants like beta carotene and vitamins A, C, and E appear to curb the damaging effects of these free radicals in the body. Very new research is finding antioxidants may also be helpful in neurological disorders such as Parkinson's and Alzheimer's disease and also in diseases like arthritis involving the immune system. Scientists are continuing to investigate how and why dietary antioxidants provide protective health benefits. In the meantime, we know antioxidant nutrients are naturally plentiful in fruits and vegetables.

Food sources of antioxidants work cooperatively. Vitamin C is a water-soluble vitamin, meaning it dissolves in water and floats around the watery inner part of the cells, scanning for free radicals and wiping them out of that area. Vitamin E, a fat-soluble vitamin, stations itself within the fat-containing cell membrane that surrounds cells, keeping that spot clean. Beta carotene appears to act efficiently in places that have what is called a low-oxygen tension, such as the capillaries of muscle tissue. The cooperative nature of antioxidants underscores the importance of eating a diet rich in vitamins. Food sources of these antioxidant vitamins are described in the next section.

MORE ABOUT VITAMIN A

Vitamin A is a generic term for compounds other than the carotenoids, which have the biologic activity of retinol. These vitamin A compounds include retinol, retinal and retinoic acid. In its natural form, vitamin A is found only in animal sources and is usually associated with fats of some type. Previtamin A, which we know as beta carotene, is the original source of retinol in plants. It is called carotene because one of its main sources is the yellow pigment in carrots. Beta carotene is the more common precursor (or beginning form of vitamin A) and supplies about two thirds of the vitamin A necessary in humans. During absorption, some of the carotene is converted to vitamin A in the intestinal wall. Vitamin A, which is fat-soluble, then is stored in our liver and fatty tissues for future use.

BETA CAROTENE

The carotenoids are a group of more than 600 related compounds widespread in nature among plants that are exposed to the sun. Of that large family of carotenoids, about 50 can be converted into vitamin A. Beta carotene is the star player in this family. Some carotenoids even carry out antioxidant activities without being converted to vitamin A.

Vitamin A content of foods and recipes in this book is expressed in retinol equivalents (RE). The Recommended Daily Allowance for Vitamin A is 800 RE for women and 1000 RE for men. One retinol equivalent equals 1 microgram (mcg.) of retinol or 6 mcg. of beta carotene.

Top Ten Vitamin A Foods	Retinol Equivalents Vitamin A
1/2 cup canned pumpkin	2691
1 baked sweet potato	2488
1 medium carrot	2025
1/2 cup mixed vegetables	995
1/2 cup cooked spinach	737
1/2 cup butternut squash	714
1/4 cantaloupe	516
1/2 cup kale	413
3 raw apricots	277
1/2 cup broccoli	110

MORE ABOUT VITAMIN C

The name ascorbic acid was given to this vitamin by its early discoverers because of its ability to fight scurvy. Vitamin C is water soluble and most unstable. It can easily be destroyed by oxygen, alkalies, and high temperatures. It also reacts with iron and copper. A concentration of vitamin C may be found in the more metabolically active tissues of the adrenal glands, brain, kidney, liver, pancreas, thymus, and spleen.

The RDA for vitamin C is 60 mg. for women and men.

Top Ten Vitamin C Foods	Milligrams of Vitamin C
1/2 cup chopped red pepper	109
1/2 medium papaya	94
1 fresh orange	80
1 raw kiwifruit	75
6 oz. orange juice from concentrate	73
1/4 cantaloupe	68
6 oz. grapefruit juice from concentrate	62
4 cooked Brussels sprouts	48
1/2 red grapefruit	47
1/2 cup strawberries	42
1/2 cup cooked broccoli	41

MORE ABOUT VITAMIN E

Vitamin E is a fat-soluble antioxidant, and its availability is far more restricted than vitamins A or C.

The requirements for vitamin E vary with the amount of polyunsaturated fatty acids in the diet. The RDA for adults is 10 milligrams alpha-tocopherol equivalents for men and 8 milligrams for women. The term alpha-tocopherol equivalents is used to measure various forms of tocopherol, the active portion of vitamin E. Food sources are the polyunsaturated vegetable oils; cottonseed, safflower, and sunflower are best.

To maximize vitamin E intake, choose among those listed above when a recipe calls for vegetable oil. In addition, there are four fruits that contribute vitamin E: apples, apricots, mangos, and pears.

VITAMIN E FOOD SOURCES	
Food	Milligrams alpha-tocopherol units
1 Tbsp. sunflower oil	6.1
1 Tbsp. cottonseed oil	4.8
1 Tbsp. safflower oil	4.6
1 oz. dried almonds	6.7
1 medium sweet potato	6.0
4 spears asparagus	1.1
1/2 cup pumpkin	0.8
1 medium raw apple	0.8
1/2 cup parsnips	0.7
1/2 cup raw green cabbage	0.6
1/2 cup turnip greens	0.6
1/2 cup raw spinach	0.5

MORE ABOUT THE CANCER CONNECTION

A simple way to visualize antioxidant activity is to imagine a police force within your body stamping out harmful effects of the contaminants and pollutants known to be the first domino in the formation of cancer. Nutrition scientists now understand these antioxidant events at the cellular level. This knowledge fits with large-scale population studies showing antioxidant-rich diets to be cancer-protective.

The Nurses' Health Study, which looked at the diets of 90,000 middle-aged women over eight years, found women whose diets were deficient in Vitamin A were at increased risk for developing breast cancer. The nurses' study group could achieve a protective level simply by eating carotene-rich foods.

More than 100 other epidemiologic studies involving large populations have found increased consumption of vegetables and fruits to be associated with a decreased cancer risk. In trying to explain these results, scientists are gaining appreciation for non-nutrients called phytochemicals. The notion that foods contain an assortment of non-nutritive components with potent biological activity is not surprising when one considers that for centuries plants and foods have been used as medicines and curative agents. Many important drugs are derived from plants. Initial interest in food phytochemicals focused largely on those found in cruciferous vegetables. But our knowledge has expanded. The National Cancer Institute's Dr. Herbert Pierson is studying these nontraditional nutrients and has identified more than 40 new substances that occur naturally in small amounts in fruits, vegetables, herbs, and grains. For instance, an orange has about 150 phytochemicals that are cancer preventing and may help lower cholesterol or act as antioxidants. The phytochemical that gives oranges their distinctive aroma, D0-limonene, may help dissolve gallstones. Among the other foods being studied are citrus fruits, garlic, soybeans, carrots, parsley, celery, and parsnips.

Other examples revealing how phytochemicals work: Allylic sulfides in garlic and onions seem to protect against stomach cancer. They work by waking up enzymes inside cells that detoxify cancer-causing chemicals. And capsaicin, which gives hot chili peppers their hot flavor, prevents carcinogens from binding to DNA, where they can trigger the changes that lead to tumor growth.

Broccoli emerged as something of a super vegetable after a group of scientists at Johns Hopkins University in Baltimore announced a sulfur-rich chemical in broccoli called sulfurophane "may be a significant component of the anticarcinogenic action of broccoli." This chemical also occurs in brussels sprouts, cauliflower, bok choy, and other members of the cruciferous family.

Cruciferous vegetables are also bursting with chemicals called indoles, which have been shown to block cancer-causing agents in animals. Results of animal trials have been striking. In one study, 68 percent of mice not receiving sulfurophane came down with breast cancer, while only 35 percent of mice receiving low does of the protective compound and a mere 26 percent of the rodents given high doses of sulfurophane contracted cancer. What is more, sulfurophane delayed the onset of the cancer and kept the number and size of any resulting tumors comparatively small. The chart on the next page summarizes additional protective benefits of phytochemicals. Keep in mind studies confirming cancer-protective benefits of the antioxidants and phytochemicals are based on real food sources, not vitamin pills or supplements.

THE PHYTOCHEMICAL PHARMACY

Food	Phytochemical	May Help Prevent
Apple	Ellagic acid	Cancer
	Octacosanol	Parkinsonism
Artichoke	Cynarin	High cholesterol
Blueberries	Anthocyanosides	Diarrhea
		Heart Disease
Celery	Psoralens	Psoriasis
Chili peppers	Capsaicin	Arthritis
		Asthma
		Bronchitis
Figs	Benzaldehyde	Cancer
		Lymphoma
Orange	D-limonene	Breast cancer
	Terpenes	Lung cancer
Pineapple	Bromelain	Cancer
		Coagulation
		Inflammation
Pumpkin	Carotenoids	Cancer
Spinach	Carotenoids	Cancer
Strawberry	Ellagic acid	Cancer
	Pectin	High cholesterol
Tomato	Lycopene	Cancer
	Gamma-aminobutyric acid	Hypertension

HOW ANTIOXIDANTS PROTECT US FROM HEART DISEASE

The first step in the development of heart disease (doctors call it coronary artery disease) involves LDL-cholesterol. Often referred to as the "bad" cholesterol, LDL-cholesterol makes its way into blood vessel walls and undergoes oxidation there. Unfortunately, once in the blood vessel walls, the oxidized LDL-cholesterol attracts other cells that contribute to the development of plaque or fatty streaks. If the plaque becomes large enough, it eventually starts to close off the vessel and causes chest pain and then a heart attack.

Scientists have theorized we can reduce the oxidation process along the blood vessel walls with antioxidants. In experiments designed to test this theory, evidence is mounting that beta carotene and vitamin E do just that. Preliminary evidence shows beta carotene even having the power to reverse the process of blood vessel clogging. The hows and whys of this process at the cellular level are continually being defined, but population studies confirm the idea. At the American Heart Association Scientific Session in November 1993, we learned women who consume high amounts of antioxidant-containing foods such as carrots and spinach had a 33 percent lower risk of heart attack and a 71 percent lower risk of stroke than women who ate few antioxidant-containing foods.

Additional news about heart disease! Trans-fatty acids, the new enemy in the war against coronary disease, are not found in fruits and vegetables. These troublesome fats are plentiful in processed foods such as margarines and vegetable shortenings. While these spreads begin as liquid vegetable oils, food manufacturers must partially load the fat molecules with hydrogen to convert them to semi-solid form. Scientists have linked trans-fatty acids to higher LDL-cholesterol (the bad kind) and lower HDL-cholesterol (the good kind). To minimize intake of these fats, choose reduced-fat or fat-free margarines or soft spreads that come in tubs. Canola, olive, and corn oils are preferred for cooking.

HOW ANTIOXIDANTS HELP FIGHT INFECTIONS

In addition to protecting blood vessels from bad cholesterol, dietary antioxidants may boost the immune system. Experts on nutrition and the immune system agree that, with the help of vitamins and minerals, older Americans may be able to recapture the immune systems they had when they were 20 years younger. Doctors have always assumed an inevitable decline in immune system with age, but that concept is being challenged.

Let's suppose a 10 year old and an 80 year old were exposed to the same cold virus. The 10 year old is sick for one day and back on his feet the next day. The older person is knocked out for a week, and it takes two weeks to fully recover. Experts are beginning to realize these so-called age-related changes in immune function are not age-related at all, but have much more to do with nutrition. In a study of 100 middle-class Canadians over the age of 65, half of the people took a multivitamin and mineral supplement with extra vitamin E and beta carotenewhile the other half took a placebo of just calcium and magnesium. The group taking the supplement had half as many colds, flus, and other infectious illnesses as the placebo group. When the study participants became sick, the supplement groups got better in half the time. Supplements were also observed to strengthen the immunity one gets from a flu vaccine. When an infection strikes, antioxidants appear to have an early repair function at the cellular level.

Antioxidants may also reduce the pain and discomfort of rheumatoid arthritis. In the diseased tissue of patients with rheumatoid arthritis, free radicals are generated in large amounts; and some studies indicate that in the presence of more antioxidants, there is less pain and less progression of the disease.

Antioxidants may also impede cataract development. Again, the oxidation process is the culprit in cataract disease. The eye lens is oxidized. Unlike other cells in the body, our lens cells are never replaced; they must last a lifetime. As we age, the lens cells become increasingly dehydrated and compressed. At the same time, the creation of free radicals alters the structure of the lens cells' protein. These clumps of protein form the cataract and effectively scatter any light coming into the eye. When the light is scattered, it cannot get through to the retina, the part of the eye responsible for sending a signal to the brain to "see something."

If oxidation creates the cataract problem, it stands to reason the antioxidant nutrients may be able to fight it. In a study of more than 1,000 people, ages 40 to 70, scientists at the State University of New York at Stony Brook found that those who had a high intake of the antioxidant nutrients had a decreased incidence of cataract formation. Further evidence: A team of scientists at Tufts University found that people who ate fewer than three and half servings of fruits and vegetables a day were eight times as likely to end up with a cataract as those who ate more. These researchers advise liberal consumption of fruits and vegetables early in life to retard the oxidation process.

HOW ANTIOXIDANTS RETARD AGING

If they are not stopped first by an antioxidant, free radicals damage body tissues. Every day millions of free radicals are formed in the body. If a few are not squelched each day, a little bit of damage begins to slowly accumulate. Over time, the accumulated damage equates with the changes of aging. Experts view higher levels of antioxidants as protective against free radicals, thus slowing the effects of aging. Animal studies confirm that after consuming supplementary doses of antioxidants in their diets, rodents have less of a certain pigment inside their cells that is associated with age.

Vitamin pills, also known as dietary supplements, cannot replace the benefits of fruits and vegetables. Natural food sources of vitamins, especially fruits and vegetables, pack the disease-preventing wallop. These plant foods harbor a whole arsenal of compounds that have never seen the inside of a vitamin bottle for the simple reason scientists have not until very recently known they even existed. Evidence from a Finnish study confirms vitamin supplements do not pack the same punch as food sources. This latest report found that after treating 29,000 male smokers with vitamin E and beta carotene supplements for five to eight years, the supplements offered no protection from cancer.

Many vitamins and minerals work best when other nutrients are present. Vitamin E improves the body's use of vitamin A. Vitamin C enhances the absorption of iron. Many of the B vitamins work together, so a deficiency of one usually affects the work of several others. Perhaps the best known nutrient interaction is that of calcium and vitamin D, which is critical for the absorption of calcium and the normal deposition of the mineral into bone.

Nature has created foods as the perfect packaging for antioxidants. And dietitians have concluded that, while supplements cause no harm, they may give a false sense of nutrition well-being and be a waste of money.

FRUITS AND VEGETABLES AND OBESITY

Vegetables and fruits are a potent aid to weight control. They are high in fiber and fill you up before you eat too many calories. A liberal intake of fruits and vegetables is the cornerstone of a low-fat diet. When we avoid fatty foods, we are less likely to store fat on our bodies, and more likely remove fat from storage for energy needs.

The sure-fire success of a low-fat diet for weight control is being tarnished by a growing number of people who overdose on low-fiber, low-sugar, but fat-free foods. Weight control specialists are seeing more and more patients with the same problem: they cannot lose weight even though they are eating a low-fat diet. The reason is often this: they have given up foods such as red meat and cheese and replaced them with reduced-fat and fat-free crackers, cheese, yogurt, cookies, cakes, frozen desserts, and other processed foods—instead of adding more fruits and vegetables. Many of these fat-free indulgences offer little satiety compared with a fiber-rich vegetable salad or fresh fruit compote, and thus total calorie intake is higher than pre-low-fat diet levels. A low-fat diet promotes weight loss only when fat-free fruits and vegetables are offered as straight replacements for higher-fat foods.

IS IT SAFE TO EAT MORE FRUITS AND VEGETABLES?

As the health benefits of fruits and vegetables add up and experts urge increased consumption, several safety issues need to be considered.

Most fruits and vegetables must be scrubbed thoroughly in cold tap water to reduce pesticide residue. An important second step in reducing pesticide exposure is to remove the outer leaves or skin of the produce before serving. Most pesticides are water-soluble and can be significantly reduced with vigorous washing. However, the Environmental Working Group recently issued a report stating that even with washing, coring, and peeling, 80 percent of peaches, apples, and celery studied contained pesticide residues. An additional study conducted at Cornell University by Dr. Nell Monday suggests potatoes should be peeled before serving. Her research detected residues from sprout inhibitors on potato peels four times greater than what government guidelines allow. Peeling the skin before boiling or steaming will keep the chemicals from migrating into the potato flesh. Likewise, discard the skin on a baked potato. Never mind vitamin losses; vitamin C is concentrated in the center of the potato, and a large, peeled potato still contributes about 2 grams of fiber. These findings are especially important for children and underscore the importance of thorough scrubbing of fresh foods.

The expanding availability of organic fruits and vegetables will be of interest to consumers who want to strictly limit exposure to pesticides. However, organically grown produce is not an immediate remedy for our concern about chemicals and pesticides in the food supply. Pesticides were created to give the human gardener the advantage and we cannot feed the masses with hand-tended produce from small farms. The Food and Drug Administration (FDA) and the Environmental Protection Agency (EPA) have built in multiple safety factors based on lifetime animal experiments to determine safe levels of pesticides in fruits and vegetables, and these are trusted by dietitians.

Genetically-altered fruits and vegetables with improved color, flavor, taste and shelf life will benefit consumers in the future. Flavr-Savr, a tomato that stays ripe longer, is now on the market and has been found by the the FDA to be as safe as tomatoes bred by conventional means. The tomato's genetic changes allow it to ripen on the vine longer, get redder, and more flavorful, and still allow growers time to ship it long distances. Genetic manipulation of vegetables is as old as human agriculture, and large scale biotechnology may be the most promising way to stop the use of chemicals in agriculture.

Biotechnology enhances many traits in plants and foods. Examples include virus-resistant melons, drought-resistant corn, higher-starch potatoes (reduces oil absorbed in frying), highly unsaturated canola oil, easy peeling oranges and grapefruit, and improved amino acid structure in beans and sunflowers.

The National Academy of Sciences, the EPA, and the FDA all have roles in the regulation of fruit and vegetable safety. They will continue to monitor pesticide levels as well as technology-driven changes in the produce supply. The strenuous efforts of these agencies lead me to believe it is safer to fill up our grocery carts at the produce section rather than roll on by it.

HOW FRUITS AND VEGETABLES FIT WITH LABELS AND PYRAMIDS

Before nutrition labeling legislation was passed in December 1992, some canned foods had no nutrition information on the label. This information must now be printed in a standard format on all canned food labels. Labeling fresh fruits and vegetables remains voluntary. Check with your produce manager for nutrient information, ot look for a flipchart presentation of fruit and vegetable labeling in the produce section of large markets.

A sample label from Del Monte® Stewed Tomatoes, Mexican Recipe is shown on the next page.

Nutrition Facts

Serving Size 1/2 cup (126 g)
Servings Per Container approx. 3 1/2

Amount Per Serving	
Calories 35	Calories from Fat 0

	% Daily Value*
Total Fat 0 g 0%	
Saturated Fat 0 g	0%
Cholesterol 0 mg	0%
Sodium 400 mg	17%
Total Carbohydrate 9 g	3%
Dietary Fiber 2 g	8%
Sugars 7 g	
Protein 1 g	
Vitamin A 10% • Vitamin C 25%	
Calcium 2% • Iron 2%	

Percent Daily Values are based on a 2,000 calorie diet.

INGREDIENTS: TOMATOES; TOMATO JUICE; SUGAR; SALT; JALAPEÑO PEPPERS; DRIED ONIONS, GREEN PEPPERS, CELERY; GARLIC POWDER; SPICES; CALCIUM CHLORIDE, CITRIC ACID.

Notice:

- Serving sizes are standarized . . . 1/2 cup for vegetables.

- Saturated fat, cholesterol, sugars, and dietary fiber per serving have joined calories, protein, fat, carbohydrate, and sodium in the nutrient listing.

- Percent Daily Value is a new term meant to give the consumer an idea of the percentage of the day's allotment of the nutrient the food provides. For instance, one serving of the tomatoes accounts for 0 percent of the recommended fat limit, but 17 percent (or 400 milligrams) of the sodium limit for a 2,000-calorie diet. If you are trying to control sodium for blood pressure concerns, an intake of 2,500 milligrams may be recommended. You may wish to find tomatoes labeled "No Added Salt" and check their sodium content.

- The B vitamins have been removed from the standard label, but antioxidants A and C are expressed in the familiar percentages of the Recommended Daily Allowance. In this case, 1/2 cup of tomatoes contributes 10 percent of vitamin A (100 RE for men, 80 RE for women) and 25 percent of vitamin C (15 milligrams for adults). Food companies may voluntarily list other vitamins as well.

- Two important minerals, calcium and iron, known to be deficient in some Americans' diets, are also noted in the nutrient panel.

Nutrient claims on fruit and vegetables may include:

- Low calorie = 40 calories or less.

- Light or Lite = 1/3 fewer calories or 50 percent less fat than regular produce. If more than half of the calories are from fat, fat content must be reduced by 50 percent or more.

- Fat-free = less than 0.5 gram of fat per serving.

- Low-fat = 3 grams or less of fat per serving.

- Cholesterol free = less than 2 milligrams cholesterol and 2 grams or less of saturated fat.

- Low cholesterol = 20 milligrams or less of cholesterol and 2 grams or less of saturated fat.

- Sodium-free = less than 5 milligrams sodium.

- High fiber = 5 grams or more fiber.

THE USDA FOOD PYRAMID

The USDA Food Pyramid, issued in 1992, calls for three to five servings of fruits and two to four servings of vegetables daily. The eating plan limits fat to 30 percent of total calorie intake. The pyramid fits the "Five-a-Day" goal and represents an increase in fruit and vegetables from the 1970s-era Daily Food Guide, which recommended four servings of fruits or vegetables daily.

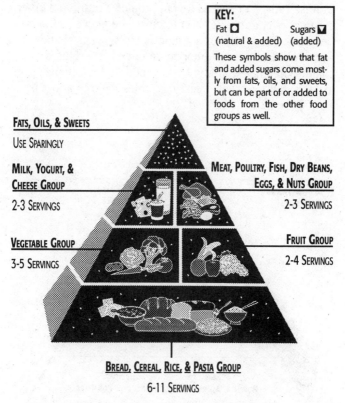

KEY:
Fat ▢ (natural & added)   Sugars ▼ (added)

These symbols show that fat and added sugars come mostly from fats, oils, and sweets, but can be part of or added to foods from the other food groups as well.

FATS, OILS, & SWEETS
USE SPARINGLY

MILK, YOGURT, & CHEESE GROUP
2-3 SERVINGS

MEAT, POULTRY, FISH, DRY BEANS, EGGS, & NUTS GROUP
2-3 SERVINGS

VEGETABLE GROUP
3-5 SERVINGS

FRUIT GROUP
2-4 SERVINGS

BREAD, CEREAL, RICE, & PASTA GROUP
6-11 SERVINGS

Source: U.S. Dept. of Agriculture/U.S. Dept. of Health and Human Services

THE MEDITERRANEAN DIET FOOD PYRAMID

Fruits and vegetables assume the same place in a newly issued Mediterranean Diet Food Pyramid. This new model for healthy eating was initiated by a group of scientists and nutritionists organized by the Harvard School of Public Health and the Oldways Preservation and Exchange Trust (a Boston-based food research organization). It is built on grains, fruits, and vegetables but promotes beans and other legumes over animal-based proteins. The plan also limits red meat to a few times per month and suggests abundant use of olive oil (rich in monounsaturated fat). This is a major difference from the USDA model which limits all types of fat. Root and green vegetables (high in antioxidants) are also emphasized.

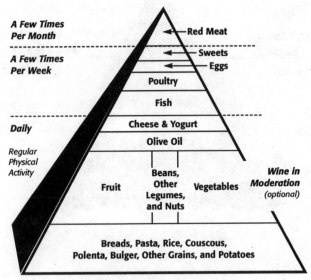

Copyright© 1994 Oldways Preservation &
Exchange Trust and Harvard School of Public Health

Preliminary evidence among heart attack survivors suggests those having had a first heart attack who then adopted a Mediterranean diet were 70 percent less likely to suffer a relapse than those following a standard low-fat diet.

What was paradise? But a garden, an orchard of trees and herbs, full of pleasure and nothing there but delights.

—William Lawson

ALL ABOUT FRUIT

So we have the idea: fruits and vegetables are good for us. Increasing our intake to five servings a day is not as drastic as it sounds. There are lots of little tricks for slipping fruit unobtrusively into the diet.

First things first—let's define a serving of fruit.

- — 1 medium apple, orange, banana, or similar-sized whole fruit
- — 1/2 cup of small or diced fruit, such as grapes or crushed pineapple
- — 1/4 cup dried fruit, such as raisins
- — 3/4 cup pure fruit juice

Fruits blend into any breakfast, lunch, or supper as sweet endings, or they may be your first choice as a snack. Choose a few new and fruity ideas from the list that follows.

- Add fresh grapes or diced apple to chicken or turkey salad from the deli.

- Keep mixed dried fruit in a plastic bag in the glovebox of the car for an instant "energy hit."

- Dilute pineapple juice with lemon-flavored mineral water for a cool drink on a hot day.

- Add 1/2 cup of dried cherries to a bran or buttermilk muffin mix that makes 12 muffins.

- Add a spoonful of all-fruit strawberry jam to nonfat cream cheese for a quick green apple dip or dice berries and top your bagels with nonfat cream cheese and berries.

- Treat your summer guests with grilled fruits; cook ripe peach or apricot wedges over medium coals, turning frequently until they are browned, and serve with grilled pork or chicken.

- Marinate leftover mixed fruits in sugar-free lemon-lime soft drink and serve over rainbow sherbet.

- Prepare a gelatin mold with a 3-ounce package of sugar-free gelatin, 1 cup water and 1 cup chopped fruit. Center the chilled mold on a plate rinsed first with cold water for perfect unmolding.

- Place dates in the freezer to ease chopping, then add them to quick bread.

- Quickly peel an orange or grapefruit by immersing the whole fruit in a pot of boiling water and letting stand for 4 minutes. Remove the fruit and peel away the skin.

- Freeze apricot nectar in an ice cube tray. Blend 3 cubes with 1 cup of any fresh fruit for a fruit frappe.

- Toss raspberries with almond or orange liqueur and serve as a topping over reduced-fat brownies.

- Got a lousy watermelon? Scoop it into balls and marinate in sugar-free strawberry soft drink and fresh mint.

- Blend any two juices together for a wonderful wake-up—apple with grape, prune with pineapple, etc.

- Use pineapple as a second topping with Canadian bacon pizza.

- Celebrate the weekend with out-of-the-ordinary fruits:

  —carambola (star fruit)
  Cut unpeeled fruit into slices, or add to fruit salads, or use as a garnish.

  —guava
  Serve plain with seeds removed, cook for compote or fill with a scoop of cottage cheese.

  —tangelos
  Peel and mix segments with sliced bananas.

- Let children create their own fruit kabobs from chunks of melon and pineapple, whole grapes, and apple, pear, and peach wedges.

- Microwave applesauce for a topping on low-fat praline frozen yogurt.

- Vary a northern diet in the winter with frozen peaches, whole raspberries, and cherries.

- Check fruit-drink labels very carefully. Look for 100 percent unsweetened fruit juice.

- Family and friends will love strawberry jam for gifts. Use Light Suregell® to minimize the sugar.

- Let children use a shaker container of cinnamon and sugar or sugar substitute to spice up tart apple slices.

- Throw blueberries into pancake batter.

- Drain liquid from juice-pack canned fruit directly into the orange-juice container.

- A mixture of hot lemon juice and honey soothes a sore throat.

- Puree odd bits of leftover fruits with a dash of sugar-free lemon gelatin for a bedtime snack.

MORE ON JUICES

While fruit juices are good for us, dietitians recommend eating whole fruits for the fiber benefit. Raw fruit and vegetable juices touted by juice machine vendors as "life-giving" are only as good as the food that goes in, and some of the nutrients are left behind in the solids. Commercial juices may be just as high in nutrients, as they are made from fruits just out of the fields, then refrigerated or frozen.

Maximize nutrition from juice by:

- looking for items that have only the word "juice" in the product name. Only products that are 100 percent pure fruit juice can call themselves simply "juice" on the label. Longer names like "fruit-juice blend" or "fruit-juice punch" or worse yet "fruit drink" indicate the product is not 100 percent juice.

- reading the ingredient label. Remember items are listed in order of weight from heaviest to lightest. If juice is listed before water or corn syrup, there is a higher percentage of real fruit juice.

- keeping juices well covered and properly chilled to conserve vitamin C.

Compare these beverage types and their real juice contents:

Fruit-juice blends	=	50 percent real juice
Fruit-juice cocktails	=	25 to 50 percent real juice
Fruit-juice punch	=	10 to 20 percent real juice
Fruit-juice drink	=	10 to 15 percent real juice
Fruit-juice beverage	=	10 to 50 percent real juice
Fruit-juice sparkler	=	70 to 80 percent real juice

THE FRESHNESS FACTOR

The vitamin C and A content of week-old produce is about the same as that of produce just out of the field. A study of the National Food Processors Association compared frozen, canned, and fresh-cooked supermarket peas, lima beans, carrots, spinach, and sweet potatoes. In the majority of cases, vitamin and mineral contents were comparable. Nutrient losses from canning or freezing produce right from the field are not much different than nutrient losses from prolonged transport and handling in fresh produce.

Fresh produce travels an average of 200 miles to reach markets. It takes a week for California broccoli to reach a Midwestern supermarket. That head of lettuce from the store has been loaded, unloaded, stored, and reloaded up to five times. Fruits and vegetables are living breathing things, secreting active enzymes and consuming their own nutrients. They are also dying things. Separated from soil and water, fruits and vegetables begin to decay. Cell walls weaken and collapse. Enzymes run rampant through the tissues and break down vitamins. The longer a fruit or vegetable sits and the more it is handled, the greater the damage.

Freshness and vitamin content are protected now by many produce managers. Wet racks are outfitted with automated mist nozzles—timed to the vegetables' need for moisture. Apples and strawberries are shipped and stored in "controlled-atmosphere" chambers that slow their respiration and extend their youth.

While some of us will continue to insist on fresh broccoli, others will be content to pour it out of the freezer bag. The idea is to realize optimal health by choosing five servings of fruits or vegetables daily—fresh, frozen, canned, dried, or juiced. Let your taste preference and need for convenience guide your selection.

FROM APPLES TO WATERMELONS: HOW TO PICK AND FIX FRUITS

Apples

The three most popular varieties are:

Red Delicious—
Bright to dark red, favorite eating apple, mildly sweet and juicy.

Golden Delicious—
Mellow, sweet, all-purpose for baking, salads, and eating; flesh stays white longer than other apples.

Granny Smith—
Green, tart, crisp, juicy; excellent for cooking, salads, and eating.

Look for: firmness with smooth, clean skin and good color. Avoid fruit with bruises or decay spots.

Fix-it tip: Prepare fresh apple dishes just before serving to minimize oxidation and browning. Once cut, apples should be dipped into a solution of one part citrus juice and three parts water or a commercial antioxidant such as Fruit Fresh®. Dissolve 1 teaspoon of Fruit Fresh in 2 tablespoons of water and use to coat fruit.

Apricots

Look for: plump fruit with as much golden orange color as possible. Blemishes, unless they break the skin, will not affect flavor. Avoid fruit that is pale yellow, greenish yellow, very firm, shriveled, or bruised. Soft, ripe fruit has the best flavor and should be used soon after purchase.

Fix-it tip: Ripen apricots at room temperature until they give to gentle pressure. To hasten ripening, group fruit in a loosely closed paper bag and check it daily. Refrigerate ripe, unwashed fruit in a paper bag for up to two days. To cut an apricot, slice around the seam and twist in half, lifting out the pit. To peel, dip in boiling water for 20 seconds. Cool quickly in cold water, then slip off the skins. Fill apricot halves with reduced-fat cream cheese and sprinkle with almonds for a quick salad or dessert.

Bananas

Look for: plump, well-filled fruit of uniform shape at desired ripeness level. Avoid produce with blemished or bruised skins. Dull grey-yellow skins indicate improper temperature maintenance, but do not mean the fruit is spoiled. Off-color bananas can be used in salads with good results.

Fix-it tip: To cut ripening time in half, place bananas in a paper bag with apples. Close the bag and let stand at room temperature. Once cut, bananas should be dipped into a solution of one part citrus juice and three parts water or a commercial antioxidant such as Fruit Fresh®. Dissolve 1 teaspoon of Fruit Fresh in 2 tablespoons of water. Use to coat fruit.

Blueberries

Look for: plump, firm berries with a light grayish bloom.

Fix-it tip: wash and serve fresh blueberries with lemon sherbet.

Cantaloupe

Look for: slightly oval fruit, 5 inches or more in diameter, with yellow or golden (not green) background color. Signs of sweetness include pronounced netting and a few tiny cracks near the stem end. Press your thumb into the stem area, it should be slightly soft. Smell the melon, it should be noticeably strong and sweet.

Fix-it tip: If not ripe, hasten ripening by placing a whole melon inside a loosely closed paper bag. Once cut, melons do not get any riper. Refrigerate cut melon in a tightly sealed plastic bag. For a pretty dish, cut off the top one fourth of a canteloupe. Hollow out the inside, using the fruit for soup. Serve the soup in the hollowed-out shell.

Cherries

Look for: plump, bright-colored sweet or sour cherries. Sweet cherries with reddish brown skin promise flavor. Avoid overly soft or shriveled cherries and those with dark stems. Cherries store best in a shallow pan, arranged in layers separated by paper towels and covered with plastic wrap.

Fix-it tip: Add sweet cherries to a chicken salad. Poach sour cherries in a small amount of grenadine and serve over vanilla frozen yogurt.

Grapefruit

Look for: firm, thin-skinned fruit, full colored, and heavy for its size. The best grapefruit are smooth, thin skinned, and flat at both ends. Avoid fruit with a pointed end or thick, deeply pored skin.

Fix-it tip: Mix fresh grapefruit sections with other fresh fruits for a sour zing sure to wake up your diners.

Grapes

Look for: plump grapes firmly attached to pliable green stems. Grapes do not sweeten or ripen after picking so color is the best indication of ripeness and flavor. Avoid soft or wrinkled fruits and those with bleached areas at the stem end.

Fix-it tip: Serve grapes with wedges of reduced-fat cheese and breadsticks for a quick appetizer.

Honeydew melon

Look for: melons weighing at least 5 pounds, with waxy white rind, barely tinged with green. Fully ripe fruit has a cream-colored rind. The blossom end should give to gentle pressure.

Fix it tip: Serve melon balls in a glass dessert dish and drizzle with Amaretto liqueur.

Kiwifruit

Look for: softness similar to a ripe peach. Choose evenly firm fruit, free of mold and soft spots. Markets usually display very firm fruit that needs to be ripened further at room temperature, uncovered, out of direct sun. Refrigerate ripe fruit in a plastic or paper bag for up to one week.

Fix-it tip: Peel a kiwi and cut into round thin slices; mix with pineapple tidbits and a fresh sliced banana for a quick fruit salad.

Lemons

Look for: firm, heavy fruit. Generally, rough-textured lemons have thicker skins and less juice than fine-skinned varieties.

Fix-it tip: Dip lemon wedges in chopped fresh parsley or in paprika for a fun garnish.

Mangoes

Look for: a fruit that gives to gentle pressure. Mangoes are usually sold quite firm and need to be ripened further before eating. Avoid those with shriveled or bruised skin. Ripen at room temperature, uncovered, out of direct sun.

Fix-it tip: Add mangoes to a spinach and fresh vegetable salad with honey-mustard dressing.

Nectarines

Look for: orange-yellow (not green) background color between areas of red. Ripe nectarines give to gentle pressure, but are not as soft as ripe peaches.

Fix-it tip: Use instead of peaches or pears for brown-bag lunches. They are less apt to bruise in transit.

Oranges

Look for: thin-skinned, firm, bright-colored fruit. Avoid oranges with any hint of softness or whitish mold at the ends.

Fix-it tip: Saute fresh orange sections with green onion and serve as a complement to pork or chicken.

Papayas

Look for: fruit with the softness of peaches and more yellow than green in the skin. Most papayas need to be ripened further after purchase in a closed brown bag at room temperature. Avoid bruised or shriveled fruit showing any signs of mold or deterioration.

Fix-it tip: Cut in half lengthwise and scoop out the seeds; or peel with a vegetable peeler and cut into slices. Sprinkle with lemon or lime juice to enhance flavor.

Peaches

Look for: creamy or yellow background color. Ripe peaches give to gentle pressure. Avoid green, extra-hard, or bruised fruit. Soft, ripe peaches can be used immediately. Peaches do not become sweeter after picking, but will soften and become juicier. Ripen firm fruit in a closed paper bag at room temperature. Store unwashed ripe fruit in the refrigerator in a paper bag for up to 3 days.

Fix-it tip: Serve fresh sliced peaches on Cream of Wheat® cereal.

Pears

Look for: clear fruit with firm skin. Pears gradually ripen after picking; thus are suited to quantity purchase. To ripen green fruit, store in a paper bag at room temperature until they give to firm pressure. Ripening takes 3 to 7 days. Refrigerate ripe pears, unwashed in a paper bag for 3 days.

Fix-it tip: Use 1 part lemon juice with 3 parts water to retard browning on cut pears. Drizzle pear slices with maple syrup and microwave on high power for 6 to 8 minutes for a hot dessert.

Pineapple

Look for: large, plump, fresh-looking fruit with green leaves and a sweet smell. Avoid fruit with soft spots, areas of decay, or fermented odor. Ripe fruit deteriorates quickly, so use shortly after purchase.

Fix-it tip: Cut pineapple lengthwise into quarters, cutting evenly through leaves and core. Use a curved knife to cut fruit from the rind, gently lifting the rind away from the core. Use the hollowed-out shell as a serving bowl for fruit salad.

Plums

Look for: fruit that is full colored. Ripe plums are slightly soft at the tip end and give when squeezed gently in the palm of the hand. Avoid fruit with broken or shriveled skin. Market plums may need to ripen a few days at room temperature.

Fix-it tip: Plums travel well in brown-bag lunches. Fill the cavity of plum halves with strawberry-flavored soft cream cheese for a simple dessert.

Raspberries

Look for: firm, plump well-shaped berries. If soft or discolored, they are overripe. Avoid baskets that looked stained from overripe berries. Use within 1 or 2 days of purchase.

Fix-it tip: Serve in a footed dessert dish with sparkling wine.

Strawberries

Look for: firm, plump berries that are full colored. Chandler, Pajaro, and Douglas varieties have excellent flavor. Chandler is preferred for freezing.

Fix-it tip: Slice strawberries onto pancakes or waffles.

Watermelon

Look for: fruit heavy for its size, well-shaped, with rind and flesh colors characteristic of their variety. Ripe melons are fragrant and slightly soft at the blossom end. Melons do not sweeten after harvest but will soften and become juicy. A melon that sloshes when shaken is probably overripe.

Three-step process for picking a winning watermelon:

1. Look first for the brightest-colored one in the bunch.

2. Next check the stem; it should be dry and brown, not green.

3. Then thump the melon with your knuckles; you should hear a low pitched sound, indicating a full juicy interior.

ALL ABOUT VEGETABLES

"I'm just not crazy about vegetables". . . a common apology from someone who grew up eating mushy, overcooked vegetables that lacked flavor or worse yet, tasted bitter. This book is here to convince such people that it's never too late to become a vegetable lover.

Let's start from the beginning. What is considered a serving of vegetables?

— 1 cup of raw leafy greens, easily fitting on a small salad plate

— 1/2 cup of other raw or cooked vegetables, about half of a broccoli spear

— 3/4 cup pure vegetable juice, just enough to fill a short glass

How to jump-start your vegetable quota:

• Drink vegetable juice cocktail instead of a soft drink when you dine out.

• Add another vegetable (such as frozen broccoli) to a can of reduced-sodium soups (such as chicken noodle soup).

- Add a vegetable (such as frozen peas) to traditional casseroles (like tuna and noodle).

- Bolster nutritional goodness of packaged rice mixes by adding a bag of California blend vegetables to it.

- Dilute your beer with tomato juice.

- Shun "naked sandwiches" and insist on added crunch, like sliced radishes or cucumbers, spinach or shredded cabbage.

- Load frozen pizza with fresh mushrooms, peppers, and onions.

- Extend chili with a second or third variety of beans, mixed vegetables, or corn.

- Stock the fridge with clear containers of raw carrots, celery, and radishes.

- Throw your favorite vegetables into some aluminum foil with reduced-fat margarine and grill alongside the burgers.

- Add a vegetable (like chunky tomatoes) to omelets or scrambled eggs.

- Serve vegetables before putting meat on the plate.

- Offer at least two servings of vegetables at the main meal of the day.

- Lace lasagna with spinach or shredded carrots.

- Add fresh peppers, mushrooms, or onions to boxed potato mixes.

- Focus on the vegetables you already enjoy, eating two spoonfuls instead of one.

- Enjoy sweet-corn season, but never add salt to the boiling water as the corn will become tough. Unsalted water will also reach a boil faster than salted water.

- Winter days call for soup on the stove. For bean soup, cook dried beans uncovered for a firm texture. Cover the pot to produce softer beans.

- No time to dice all those veggies for stir-fry? Go ahead and buy the frozen stir-fry blend. Add to the wok or skillet during the last 3 minutes of cooking, cover and steam until tender.

- Don't feel guilty about plain old canned green beans for the kids' lunch. It's a start in the right direction.

- Add one of those dry packaged vegetable soup mixes to 1 cup reduced-fat mayonnaise and 1 cup nonfat sour cream for a party dip.

- Need entertainment for a picnic? Kids of all ages love to spit watermelon seeds.

- Extend your favorite brand of salsa during the tomato season by adding 1 cup of chopped seeded fresh tomatoes to a 12 oz. jar.

- It's OK to add bits of leftover bacon to asparagus, brussels sprouts, or green beans.

FROM ARTICHOKES TO ZUCCHINI— HOW TO PICK AND FIX VEGETABLES

Artichokes

Look for: tight compact heads that feel heavy for their size. Surface brown spots do not affect quality.

Fix-it tip: Clean just before cooking. Using a stainless steel knife, slice off the stem. Remove and discard coarse outer leaves, then cut off the top third of the artichoke. Snip off thorny tips of remaining leaves with kitchen shears. Rinse well and plunge immediately into a solution of 1 part lemon juice to 3 parts water to prevent browning. In a large, deep pan, boil 1 gallon water, 1/4 cup vinegar, 1 tablespoon salad oil, 10 peppercorns, and 2 bay leaves. Add 5 artichokes and return to a boil. Cover and boil for 30 minutes until the stem end is tender when pierced; drain and serve with a dipping sauce. Melt 3 parts reduced-fat margarine with 1 part lemon juice and 1 part fresh chives or parsley; or dip in freshly grated Parmesan cheese.

Asparagus

Look for: firm, brittle spears that are bright green almost their entire length, with tightly closed tips. Wrap ends in a damp paper towel and refrigerate unwashed for up to three days.

Fix-it tip: Add chopped asparagus to omelets or serve cooked, chilled asparagus with your favorite oil and vinegar or Italian salad dressing.

Beans, Green or Wax

Look for: slender, crisp beans that are bright and blemish-free. Avoid mature beans with large seeds and swollen pods. Refrigerate, unwashed, in a plastic bag for up to four days.

Fix-it tip: Dress up cooked green beans with dill weed and crumbled bacon.

Beets

Look for: firm, smooth-skinned, small to medium beets. Leaves should be deep green and fresh looking. Cut off the tops leaving 1 inch of stem attached. Refrigerate for up to a week.

Fix-it tip: Scrub before cooking, but do not peel. Leave roots, stems, and skin intact. Try wrapping beets in foil and baking in the oven for 1 hour at 400°; then peel, slice, and serve with grated orange peel and nonfat sour cream.

Bok Choy

Look for: heads with bright white stalks and glossy dark leaves. Avoid heads with slippery brown spots on the leaves. Use as soon as possible after purchase.

Fix-it tip: Cut leaves from the stalks, slice the stalks cross-wise and coarsely shred the leaves for steaming. Drizzle with reduced-sodium teriyaki sauce and serve as a side dish with grilled meats.

Broccoli

Look for: compact clusters of tightly closed dark green florets. Avoid heads with yellow florets or thick, woody stems.

Fix-it tip: Rinse and cut off base of stalk. Cut into spears, cover, and microcook on high power with 2 tablespoons of orange juice and 1 teaspoon for rosemary for 3 to 5 minutes or until tender-crisp.

Brussels Sprouts

Look for: firm, compact, fresh-looking sprouts that are bright green. They should feel heavy for their size. Pull off and discard any limp leaves, then refrigerate, unwashed for three days.

Fix-it tip: To ensure even cooking, cut a shallow "X" in the stem ends of sprouts. Steam and season with basil and finely grated lemon rind.

Cabbage

Look for: firm heads that feel heavy for their size. Outer leaves should have good color and be free of blemishes. Refrigerate unwashed cabbage for up to 10 days.

Fix-it tip: Use shredded cabbage to add texture to any fresh salad; or cut it into chunks, steam, and season with caraway seed and brown sugar.

Carrots

Look for: firm, clean, well-shaped carrots with bright orange-gold color. Carrots with their tops still attached are likely to be freshest.

Fix-it tip: Cut into coins, steam, and season with nutmeg.

Cauliflower

Look for: firm, compact creamy-white heads with florets pressed tightly together. A yellow tinge and spreading florets indicate overmaturity. Leaves should be crisp and bright green.

Fix-it tip: Remove and discard outer leaves, and cut out the core. Place whole head, stem side down, in a microwave-safe bowl, add 2 tablespoons of water, and microcook on high power for 10 minutes. Sprinkle reduced-fat cheese over the top and garnish with paprika.

Celery

Look for: crisp, rigid green stalks with fresh-looking leaves. Avoid celery with limp stalks. Refrigerate, unwashed, for up to two weeks.

Fix-it tip: Add chopped celery to almost any other vegetable to extend it. Try tarragon for a complementary seasoning.

Corn

Look for: fresh-looking ears with green husks, moist stems, and silk ends free of decay or worm injury. When pierced with a thumbnail, kernels should give a squirt of juice. Tough skins indicate overmaturity. Wrap unhusked ears in damp paper towels and refrigerate in a plastic bag for up to two days.

Fix-it tip: Peel the husk back and remove the silk, then replace the husk to enclose the kernels completely. Place in the center of the microwave oven and cook on high power for 2 minutes per ear. Rearrange ears halfway through cooking. Let stand for 3 minutes, then peel husks and serve with chili powder.

Cucumbers

Look for: firm, dark green slicing, pickling, or greenhouse cucumbers that are slender but well-shaped. Soft or yellow cukes are overmature. Refrigerate whole or cut cucumbers in a plastic bag for up to a week.

Fix-it tip: Cucumbers are waxed to preserve moisture. Peel waxed cucumbers with a vegetable peeler. Use sliced cukes instead of lettuce to add crunch to sandwiches.

Eggplant

Look for: firm eggplant that is heavy for its size, with taut, glassy, deeply colored skin. The stem should be bright green. Dull skin and rust-colored spots are signs of age. Refrigerate, unwashed, in a plastic bag for up to five days.

Fix-it tip: Cut off stem, peel, and then cut eggplant into 1/2-inch-thick slices. Arrange slices on a baking sheet, brush all sides with reduced-fat Italian salad dressing, and bake in a 450° oven for 15 minutes, until tender.

Greens

Look for: fresh, tender leaves that are free of blemishes. Dark leafy greens have a pronounced flavor. Varieties include beet greens, collards, dandelion greens, kale, mustard, and turnip greens. Avoid bunches with thick, coarse-veined leaves.

Fix-it tip: Tear out and discard tough stems and center ribs. Cover coarsely chopped leaves with water and boil for 10 minutes or until tender. Serve with oregano, wine vinegar, and crumbled bacon.

Jicama

Look for: firm, well-formed tubers, free of blemishes. Size does not affect flavor, but larger roots do tend to have a coarse texture. Store whole, unwashed jicama in a cool, dark, dry place for up to three weeks. Wrap cut pieces in plastic and refrigerate for up to a week.

Fix-it tip: Scrub well and peel with a knife. Cut into julienne strips and serve with a dip or add to green salads.

Kolrabi

Look for: young, tender bulbs with fresh green leaves. Avoid those with scars and blemishes. The smaller the bulb, the more delicate the flavor and texture. Cut off leaves and stems. Refrigerate unwashed for up to a week.

Fix-it tip: Scrub well and peel. Serve kolrabi raw on a relish plate, use instead of cabbage in salad recipes, or cut into chunks and add to stews and soups during the last 20 minutes of cooking.

Leeks

Look for: leeks with clean white bottoms and crisp, fresh-looking green tops. Refrigerate, unwashed, in a plastic bag for up to a week.

Fix-it tip: Cut off and discard root ends. Trim the tops, leaving about 3 inches of green leaves. Strip away and discard coarse outer leaves, leaving tender inner ones. Wash and trim leeks under cold running water, separating layers carefully to rinse out any dirt. Add sliced leeks to chicken soups and stews or cook with carrots or peas for variety. Tarragon is a complementary seasoning.

Mushrooms

Look for: blemish-free mushrooms without slimy spots or signs of decay. Wrap in paper towels and refrigerate unwashed in a plastic bag for up to five days.

Fix-it tip: Wipe mushrooms with a damp cloth to remove dirty residue. Slice thin and add to the top of grilled meats during the last several minutes of cooking.

Okra

Look for: small to medium pods that are deep-green and free of blemishes. Pods should snap or puncture easily with slight pressure. Refrigerate, unwashed, in a plastic bag for up to 5 days.

Fix-it tip: Avoid cooking okra in iron, tin, copper, or brass pans as these metals cause discoloration. Add to gumbo dishes during the last 20 minutes of cooking.

Onions

Look for: green onions (also called scallions) with crisp, bright green tops and clean, white bottoms. Choose firm, dry onions with brittle outer skin, avoiding those with sprouting green shoots or dark spots. Refrigerate green, unwashed onions in a plastic bag for up to 10 days. Store dry unwrapped onions in a dry, cool, dark place with good ventilation for up to 2 months. Wrap cut pieces in plastic wrap and refrigerate for up to 4 days.

Fix-it tip: Peel medium-size dry onions and stand upright in a baking dish. Bake for 30 minutes, uncovered, in a 350° oven and baste with reduced-fat margarine and finely-grated orange rind.

Parsnips

Look for: small to medium parsnips that are smooth, firm and well shaped. Avoid large roots because they are likely to have a woody core. Refrigerate, unwashed, in a plastic bag for up to two weeks.

Fix-it tip: Trim and discard the tops and root ends. Peel with a vegetable peeler, then rinse. Leave whole or dice, shred, or cut into julienne strips. Bake chopped parsnips with chunks of cooking apple in brown sugar and apple juice.

Peas

Look for: small, plump, bright green pods that are firm, crisp, and well-filled. Refrigerate, unwashed, in a plastic bag for up to 5 days.

Fix-it tip: Top steamed peas with finely shredded fresh mint. Use snap peas as a fresh vegetable dipper.

Peppers

Look for: bright glossy peppers that are firm and well shaped. Avoid those with soft spots or gashes. Refrigerate, unwashed, in a plastic bag for up to a week.

Fix-it tip: Saute red and yellow peppers and add to rice, barley, or pasta side dishes.

Potatoes

Look for: firm, smooth potatoes with no wrinkles, sprouts, cracks, bruises, decay, or bitter green areas (caused by exposure to light). Store in a cool, dark, well-ventilated area, not in an airtight plastic bag or container.

Fix-it tip: To preserve whiteness, cover peeled potatoes with cold water for a short time before cooking. Use baked potatoes as a quick supper. Put a variety of toppings on the table—cottage cheese, reduced-fat ranch dressing, chopped ham or turkey, shredded reduced-fat cheeses, chopped onion or pepper, nonfat sour cream, bacon bits, and salsa.

Rutabagas

Look for: small to medium rutabagas that are smooth, firm, and heavy for their size. Store unwrapped in a cool, dry, dark place with good ventilation for up to 2 months.

Fix-it tip: Rinse and peel with a vegetable peeler. Leave whole or slice for cooking; mash cooked rutabagas and season with brown sugar and cinnamon.

Salad greens

Look for: crisp, fresh-looking, deeply colored leaves, free of brown spots, yellowed leaves, and decay. Heads of lettuce should give a little under pressure. Choose from arugula, Belgian endive, butterhead lettuce, chicory, escarole, iceberg lettuce, looseleaf lettuce, radicchio, romaine lettuce, spinach, and watercress for salad variety. Rinse greens with cold water, shake off excess, and dry well. Wrap in paper towels and refrigerate up to 1 week. Tear salad greens into bite-size pieces.

Fix-it tip: Combine greens with leftover cooked vegetables and meat, add a reduced-fat dressing, and you have a main dish salad.

Summer Squash

Look for: yellow squash and zucchini of medium size with firm, smooth, glossy, tender skin. Squash should feel heavy for their size. Refrigerate, unwashed, in a plastic bag for up to five days.

Fix-it tip: Place slices of squash on a baking pan, brush with oil and vinegar dressing, sprinkle with grated Parmesan, and broil for 5 minutes until tender.

Sweet Potatoes and Yams

Look for: firm well-shaped vegetables with bright, uniformly colored skin. Store in a cool, dry, dark, well-ventilated place for up to 2 months.

Fix-it tip: Bake sweet potatoes and top with brown sugar and grated orange peel.

Tomatoes

Look for: smooth, well-formed tomatoes that are firm, but not hard. Store unwashed tomatoes at room temperature, stem end down until slightly soft.

Fix-it tip: To peel, submerge tomatoes in boiling water for 30 seconds, then lift out and plunge into cold water.

When cool, slip off skins. For either peeled or unpeeled tomatoes, cut out core. To seed, cut in half crosswise and squeeze out the seeds. Chop fresh tomatoes, season with salt, pepper, and minced cilantro.

Turnips

Look for: firm, smooth, small to medium-size turnips that feel heavy for their size. Remove the tops if desired; cook tops separately. Refrigerate, unwashed, in a plastic bag for up to a week.

Fix-it tip: Rinse and peel, then cube, slice, quarter, or leave whole. Serve thinly sliced raw turnips as a vegetable dipper. Season hot cooked turnips with dill.

Winter Squash

Look for: hard, thick-shelled squash. Store whole squash unwrapped in a cool, dry, dark place with good ventilation for up to two months.

Fix-it tip: Season cooked acorn or butternut squash with allspice, cardamom, cinnamon, or nutmeg.

COOKING FRESH VEGETABLES

When boiling vegetables, use just enough water to keep the pot from scorching. Better yet, use a steamer. Less contact with cooking water means less leaching of water-soluble nutrients—the B and C vitamins. Bring the water to a boil before dropping in the vegetables. Be sure lids fit tightly. Cook till just tender, not mushy. Vitamins C and B_6 are more likely to be lost during long, slow, wet cooking and conserved when cooking is quick, hot, and dry—such as stir-frying. Slice vegetables just before cooking, or cook them whole or in big chunks and cut them afterwards. Slicing and dicing expose the inner surfaces to air, allowing vitamins A and C to oxidize more rapidly. Boil-in-the-bag and microwave varieties of frozen vegetables have an advantage. Microcooking preserves nutrients by reducing cooking time and leaching.

DAILY MENUS
FEATURING FIVE OR MORE SERVINGS
OF FRUITS AND VEGETABLES DAILY

Check index for page number of featured recipes

Monday

Breakfast
Orange-pineapple juice
Bran flakes with fresh banana sliced on top
1 percent milk
Blueberry muffin from a mix with an extra 1/2 cup dried
    cherries thrown in
Coffee

Lunch
*Ham and Bean Soup
Italian breadsticks
*Spinach Salad with Blue Cheese Dressing
*Frozen Apricot Cups
Strawberry iced tea

Dinner
Fast-food takeout:
Grilled chicken breast sandwich with lettuce, pickles
    and tomato
Side salad with reduced-fat dressing
Low-fat frozen yogurt cone
Orange juice

Snacks through the day
Assorted fresh vegetables with *Classic Dill Dip
*Fresh Tomato Cocktail
Toasted white bagels with nonfat cream cheese and
    orange marmalade

Tuesday

Breakfast
Grape juice
Raisin French toast with syrup and diced peaches
Lean grilled ham
Hot tea

Lunch
Brown bag in the car:
Roast beef on rye sandwich with brown mustard and
    cucumber slices
Reduced-fat potato chips
Fresh baby carrots
Granny Smith apple
Canned pineapple-orange juice

Dinner
Grilled pork chops
*Fresh Peas with Sugar and Spice
*Fruity Parsnips
Cracked-wheat bread
Dried or canned tropical fruit mix over low-fat
    frozen yogurt

Snacks through the day
*Spiced Cider
Pretzels with reduced-fat soft cheddar cheese for dipping
Mixed dried apricots and pineapple

Wednesday

Breakfast
Cream of Wheat® with 1 percent milk and
    fresh raspberries
Bran muffin from a mix with 1/2 cup chopped dates
    thrown in
Coffee

Lunch
*Calico Bean Casserole
Broiled French bread with fresh Parmesan sprinkled on top
*Seven-Layer Salad
Cranberry-raspberry juice

Dinner
*Shepherd's Pie
*Green Beans Provencale
Crusty Italian rolls with reduced-fat margarine
*Country Apple Delight
1 percent milk

Snacks through the day
Dried pineapple over lemon sherbet
*Creamy Papaya Cooler
Watermelon balls marinated in sugar-free lemonade

Thursday

Breakfast
Apricot nectar
Cinnamon rolls from a tube with
    1/4 cup dried cranberries rolled in
Poached egg
Coffee

Lunch
Clean out leftover fruits from the week, chop and mix
    with 1 percent cottage cheese
Reduced-fat wheat crackers
*Cucumber Carrot Salad
Hot tea

Dinner
*Gazpacho
*Vegetable burritos
Chopped lettuce, peppers, onions and tomatoes on the side
*Marinated Pears
1 percent milk

Snacks through the day
Spicy hot vegetable juice cocktail
Crunchy breadsticks with string cheese
Reduced-fat yellow cupcake sliced with fresh strawberries
    and non-fat yogurt on top

Friday

Breakfast
*Snap Out Of It!
Toaster waffles with syrup and sliced kiwifruit
Broiled bacon
Low-fat fruited yogurt
Coffee

Lunch
*Stir-fry Vegetable and Wild Rice Salad
Onion bagel with reduced-fat cheddar cheese
Fresh orange
1 percent milk

Dinner
Out on the town:
Red wine (1 glass)
Grilled sirloin with peppers and mushrooms
Baked potato with sour cream
Tossed greens and mixed vegetable salad with
    reduced-fat dressing
Tomato juice

Snacks through the day
*Vegetable Pizza Squares
Prune juice laced with sugar-free lemon-lime soft drink
Bing cherries

Saturday

Late breakfast
Orange juice
Scrambled eggs with okra and yellow peppers
Hashbrowns with green onions, pan-grilled with
    reduced-fat margarine
Wheat toast with strawberry preserves
Coffee

Afternoon snack
*Choose-Your-Passion Stuffed Celery
1 percent milk

Company for dinner
*Sparkling Punch (for a wine punch, add 1 part sparkling
    white wine to 2 parts punch)
*Eggplant Dip for French Bread
*Stuffed Peppers Italiano
*Vegetable Kabobs on the Grill
Corn bread from a mix with 1/4 cup green chilies
    thrown in
*Orange Berry Cream
Hazelnut cream decaf coffee

Sunday

Brunch
Cran-grape juice mixed with sugar-free gingerale
*Mex-i-skins
Baked egg casserole with lean ham and asparagus
*Sandy's Spinach and Apple Salad
*Lemon Fruit Dip with assorted fruit dippers
Coffee

Afternoon snack
*Pears and Berries Soup
Vanilla wafers

Early dinner
*Ranch Dip with Fresh Vegetable Dippers
Grilled turkey breast with barbecue sauce
*Cauliflower with Cheese Sauce
*Western Sweet Potato Salad
White rolls with reduced-fat margarine
*Blueberries with Pecan Sauce
Hot tea

SCRIBBLES FROM THE RECIPE TESTING NOTEBOOK:

1. The recipes that follow generally call for whole amounts of fresh produce, such as 1 large onion or 1 bunch broccoli. I have used this method to save you precious minutes in the kitchen by minimizing the need to measure or wash measuring devices.

2. Where brand names are used, I have tested the recipe with that product and recommend it.

3. Adding dressing to salads is always a matter of personal taste. Some folks like their salad relatively dry . . . while others want every bite dripping. If you have leftover dressing in the shaker container, refrigerate it for up to a week for a second salad.

4. When recipes list options for egg or sugar substitutes, nutrient analysis for both is given.

5. If green onions are called for, it's OK to substitute 1/4 cup chopped yellow or white onion for each green onion.

6. Salt is minimized in the recipes. If you have no problem with high blood pressure, additional salt may safely please your palate.

7. Nutrient analysis of whole recipes yields calorie values per serving. From there, grams of fat, carbohydrate and protein are calculated. Grams are then rounded to whole numbers. If a serving has less than half a gram of fat, 0 fat is listed.

8. Published records of the vitamin content of fruits and vegetables vary widely. This is because three samples of carrots from three different locations may all yield different amounts of vitamin A. The bibliography lists my nutrient analysis sources. Try not to get lost in the fine print.

9. Recipes for fruits and vegetables fit nicely with food plans for weight control and diabetes. A "food exchange" value is included for each recipe and is based on the Exchange List for Meal Planning, a system developed and published by the American Dietetic Association and the American Diabetes Association. This system places foods into six groups with foods in each group having about the same nutritive value. The groups include bread/starch, meat, vegetable, fruit, skim milk, and fat. The system is similar to that of Weight Watchers International.

10. Vitamin E values greater than half a milligram alpha-tocopherol units per serving are noted with specific oils tested. In most cases, sunflower oil was used because it has the greatest concentration of vitamin E.

REFERENCES

1. American Cancer Society. Cancer facts and figures. Atlanta: American Cancer Society, 1993.

2. Doll, R. The causes of cancer: quantitative estimates and avoidable risks of cancer in the United States today. Journal of the National Cancer Institute. 1991; 66:1193-1309.

3. Division of Cancer Prevention and Control. Five A Day for Better Health: A Baseline Study of American's Fruit and Vegetable Consumption. National Cancer Institute and National Institutes of Health, 1992.

4. Putnam, J. Agricultural Economist. U.S. Government Economic Research Service. Scripps Howard News Service, December, 1992.

5. Pennington, J. Food Values of Portions Commonly Used. City: New York: Harper Perennial, 1994.

6. Nurses Health Study. New England Journal of Medicine. 1993; vol. 323 p. 1444-9 .

7. Will designer foods fortified with phytochemicals fight cancer? Environmental Nutrition. 1993 ; vol 16 No. 3.

8. Talalay, P. Sulforaphane Halts tumor growth. Proceedings of the National Academy of Sciences, April, 1994

9. Duke, J. The Phytochemical Pharmacy. Washington, D.C.: USDA, 1993.

10. Trans-fatty acids: The new enemy. Harvard Heart Letter. July 1994.

11. Blumberg, J.: Can Taking Supplements Help You Ward Off Disease?: Tufts University Diet and Nutrition Letter. April 1991: 9:2.

12. Peel your potatoes to avoid toxins. Environmental Nutrition. February 1993, p. 8.

BIBLIOGRAPHY

American Dietetic Association and American Diabetes Association. Exchange Lists for Meal Planning. Chicago, 1986.

Anderson, J. Plant Fiber in Foods. Lexington, KY: HCF Nutrition Research Foundation, Inc., 1990.

Elving, P.: Fresh Produce. Menlo Park, CA: Lane Publishing Co., 1987

Lyon Cardiovascular Hospital: Mediterranean diet. Lancet. 1994; June 11.

Nutra-Calc. Nutrient analysis software for Macintosh computers. Camde Corporation. 1994.

Pesticide found in scrubbed food. Washington Post. May 20, 1994, 8A

Plantation Baking Company. Survey of Midwest elementary schoolchildren. 1994.

Ziegler, R.G. Vegetables, fruits and carotenoids and the risk of cancer. American Journal of Clinical Nutrition. pp. 251S-259S, 1991.

APPETIZERS

APRICOT DIP FOR FRUITS

8 servings, 1/4 cup each

2/3 cup reduced-fat mayonnaise
2/3 cup plain nonfat yogurt
1/2 cup all-fruit apricot preserves
2 tsp. finely grated orange rind
Garnish: twisted orange slices

Combine all ingredients in a serving bowl and mix well.
Garnish the bowl with a twisted orange slice. Serve as a
dip with melon wedges, whole strawberries, pineapple
chunks, and fresh grapes.

121 calories, 6 gm. fat, 1 gm. protein, 14 gm. carbohydrate,
0 cholesterol, 152 mg. sodium, 0.4 gm. dietary fiber,
34 RE vitamin A, 4 mg. vitamin C, 0 vitamin E as alpha tocopherol

Food exchange
1 1/2 fruit, 1 fat

Preparation time
10 minutes

ARTICHOKES STUFFED IN A PITA

8 servings, 1/2 pita each

1 Tbsp. vegetable oil
1 small onion, finely chopped
1/2 tsp. garlic powder
5 oz. canned artichoke hearts, well drained
4 small tomatoes, chopped and seeds removed
3 Tbsp. minced fresh parsley
3 Tbsp. cider vinegar
4 pita bread, cut in half
Garnish: 2 oz. feta cheese, broken into pieces

Heat oil in a skillet. Saute onion, garlic powder and artichoke hearts until onion is translucent. Add tomatoes, parsley, and vinegar. Heat through. Stuff hot vegetable mixture into pita bread. Garnish the with feta cheese, and serve.

146 calories, 3 gm. fat, 5 gm. protein, 23 gm. carbohydrate, 6 mg. cholesterol, 275 mg. sodium, 1.4 gm. dietary fiber, 44 RE vitamin A, 15 mg. vitamin C, 0 vitamin E as alpha tocopherol

Food exchange
2 vegetable, 1 bread/starch, 1/2 fat

Preparation time
20 minutes

BLUE CHEESE DIP FOR APPLES

8 servings, 1/2 cup of fruit and 1/4 cup of dip each

4 oz. reduced-fat cheddar cheese, shredded
4 oz. blue cheese, crumbled
3 oz. nonfat cream cheese, softened
3 Tbsp. grated onion
1 Tbsp. Worcestershire sauce
2 Tbsp. chopped pecans or walnuts
2 large Granny Smith apples
2 large Red Delicious apples
2 Tbsp. lemon juice
1/2 cup water

In a small mixing bowl, combine first four ingredients. Mix until smooth. Spread mixture over an oval-shaped platter, about 8 to 10 inches long. Sprinkle nuts over cheese. Core apples and slice into thin wedges. In a small mixing bowl, combine lemon juice and water. Dip apples in the lemon juice bath to prevent browning. Drain apples well, then place slices on top of the nuts, fan style, down the length of the platter. Serve with a spoon, dipping some cheese with each apple slice.

178 calories, 11 gm. fat, 9 gm. protein, 12 gm. carbohydrate, 24 mg. cholesterol, 368 mg. sodium, 1.4 gm. dietary fiber, 89 RE vitamin A, 3 mg. vitamin C, 0.6 mg. vitamin E as alpha tocopherol

Food exchange
1 skim milk, 1/2 fruit, 1 1/2 fat

Preparation time
20 minutes

CHEESE-STUFFED PRUNES

No use for appetizers? This recipe makes a tasty accompaniment to a bowl of soup for a winter supper.

8 servings, 4 prunes each

4 oz. reduced-fat cheddar cheese, shredded
3 Tbsp. diced green chilies
2 Tbsp. chopped pecans
2 Tbsp. nonfat sour cream or yogurt
12 oz. pitted prunes

Preheat broiler. Combine cheese, chilies, pecans, and sour cream in a bowl; mix to blend thoroughly. Set aside. Split the prunes and form a pouch. Fill generously with cheese mixture. Place on a baking sheet and broil for 2 minutes until the cheese begins to melt. Dried apricots may be used instead of prunes.

181 calories, 5 gm. fat, 6 gm. protein, 28 gm. carbohydrate, 10 mg. cholesterol, 116 mg. sodium, 2.2 gm. dietary fiber, 135 RE vitamin A, 1 mg. vitamin C, 0 vitamin E as alpha tocopherol

Food exchange
1 1/2 fruit, 1 fat, 1/2 skim milk

Preparation time
20 minutes

Broiling time
2 minutes

CHEESY SPINACH ROLLS

8 servings, 4 rolls each

2 10 - oz. pkg. frozen spinach, thawed and
   squeezed dry
1 1/2 cup low-fat cottage cheese, drained well
1/2 cup Parmesan cheese
1/2 cup chopped red onion
2 Tbsp. chopped fresh dill or 2 tsp. dried dill weed
1 tsp. Tabasco® sauce
1/4 tsp. salt
2 tubes refrigerated pizza crust dough

Preheat oven to 375° F. Combine first seven ingredients in
a medium mixing bowl. Remove pizza crust dough from
tube and roll out flat. Spread half of the spinach and
cheese mixture on each crust. Roll up in jelly roll fashion
and seal edges of crust. Bake for 20 to 22 minutes until
crust is evenly brown. Cool for 10 minutes; slice and serve.

287 calories, 7 gm. fat, 16 gm. protein, 40 gm. carbohydrate, 7 mg.
cholesterol, 522 mg. sodium, 1 gm. dietary fiber, 550 RE vitamin A,
9 mg. vitamin C, 0.5 mg. vitamin E as alpha tocopherol

Food exchange
2 bread/starch, 2 vegetable, 1 1/2 lean meat

Preparation time
15 minutes

Baking time
22 minutes

Cooling time
10 minutes

CHOOSE-YOUR-PASSION STUFFED CELERY

8 servings, 1 full rib (3 pieces) each

1 bunch celery (about 8 ribs)

Passion-for-Cream-Cheese Filling:

3 oz. nonfat cream cheese
2 Tbsp. chopped almonds
2 Tbsp. crushed pineapple, well drained
1/4 tsp. seasoned salt
2 tsp. finely grated onion

Passion-for-Crab Filling:

6 oz. crab meat, well drained and flaked fine
1/2 cup reduced-fat mayonnaise
2 Tbsp. catsup
1 tsp. horseradish
1 Tbsp. pickle relish
3 drops Tabasco® sauce

Passion-for-Guacamole Filling:

1 ripe avocado, mashed smooth with a fork
2 tsp. lemon juice
1/4 tsp. seasoned salt
1/4 tsp. garlic powder
1/4 tsp. white pepper
1/4 cup reduced-fat mayonnaise

Wash celery and remove but save the leaves on stalks. Dry celery thoroughly before stuffing. Choose your favorite filling and combine all ingredients in a small mixing bowl. Stuff the ribs and then cut in thirds for serving. Arrange on a bed of celery leaves.

Passion-for-Cream-Cheese:
35 calories, 2 gm. fat, 3 gm. protein, 1 gm. carbohydrate,
0 cholesterol, 16 mg. sodium, 1.7 gm. dietary fiber, 16 RE vitamin A,
0 vitamin C, 1.7 mg. vitamin E as alpha tocopherol

Food exchange
1/2 skim milk

Passion-for-Crab:
38 calories, 1 gm. fat, 4 gm. protein, 4 gm. carbohydrate
18 mg. cholesterol, 284 mg. sodium, 0.9 gm. dietary fiber,
5 RE vitamin A, 2 mg. vitamin C, 0 vitamin E as alpha tocopherol

Food exchange
1 lean meat

Passion-for-Guacamole:
52 calories, 3 gm. fat, 2 gm. protein, 4 gm. carbohydrate,
0 cholesterol, 127 mg. sodium, 0.8 gm. dietary fiber,
20 RE vitamin A, 4 mg. vitamin C, 0 vitamin E as alpha tocopherol

Food exchange
1 vegetable, 1/2 fat

Preparation time
15 minutes

CLASSIC DILL DIP FOR VEGETABLES

8 servings, 1/4 cup each

1 cup reduced-fat mayonnaise
1 cup nonfat sour cream
2 Tbsp. dry onion soup mix
1 Tbsp. dried dill weed
Assorted fresh vegetables for dipping

For something different, try strips of yellow squash, aspara-gus tips, red pepper rings, radish roses, broccoli flower tops, whole fresh pea pods and whole baby carrots.

In a small mixing bowl, combine first four ingredients. Cover and refrigerate at least 30 minutes. Serve with fresh vegetables. This dip stays fresh for up to five days.

69 calories, 2 gm. fat, 2 gm. protein, 9 gm. carbohydrate, 0 cholesterol, 315 mg. sodium, 0 dietary fiber, 151 RE vitamin A, 0 vitamin C, 0 vitamin E as alpha tocopherol

Food exchange
1/2 bread/starch, 1/2 fat

Preparation time
20 minutes

Chilling time
20 minutes

EGGPLANT DIP FOR FRENCH BREAD

8 servings, 1/2 cup each

1 large eggplant
1 Tbsp. tomato juice
1 Tbsp. vegetable oil
1 green pepper, diced
2 ribs celery, diced
1 onion, diced
1 carrot, finely shredded
1/4 tsp. garlic powder
2 Tbsp. cider vinegar
1 large tomato, peeled, seeded, and chopped
1 Tbsp. basil

Cut eggplant in half lengthwise. Scoop out the pulp, leaving 1/2 to 3/4 inch shell. Reserve the pulp. Brush inside of eggplant shell with tomato juice to retard browning. Place the reserved pulp in a microwave-safe dish. Add 1 table-spoon of water and cover. Micro-cook for 8 minutes. Meanwhile, heat the oil in a skillet. Saute green pepper, celery, onion and carrot for 4 minutes. Stir in garlic powder, vinegar, tomato, and basil. Add cooked pulp and heat through. Stuff pulp mixture back into the eggplant shell. Serve as a hot dip with chunks of French bread.

55 calories, 1 gm. fat, 1 gm. protein, 9 gm. carbohydrate,
0 cholesterol, 22 mg. sodium, 1.8 gm. dietary fiber, 286 RE vitamin
A, 32 mg. vitamin C, 0 vitamin E as alpha tocopherol

Food exchange
2 vegetable

Preparation time
20 minutes

ELEGANT HOT VEGGIE APPETIZER

8 servings, 1 cup vegetable and 1 oz. dip

4 yellow squash, washed, trimmed, and sliced
  1/2-inch thick
1 lb. fresh asparagus, washed and trimmed
1 medium head cauliflower, washed and cut
  into florets
1 medium bunch broccoli, washed and cut
  into florets
1 pint cherry tomatoes
4 oz. reduced-fat Swiss cheese, shredded
1 tsp. prepared mustard
1 tsp. dill seed
1/4 cup reduced-fat cream cheese
1 Tbsp. skim milk

Arrange slices of squash around the edges of a microwave-safe platter. Next lay the asparagus spears down the middle of the platter. Arrange the broccoli and cauliflower florets around the asparagus on both sides. Sprinkle the platter with 1 Tbsp. of water and cover tightly with plastic food wrap. Microcook on high power for 4 minutes. Meanwhile, in a decorative microwave-safe dish, mix together remaining ingredients for a Swiss-cheese dip.

When vegetables are finished steaming, remove from the microwave, leaving the plastic wrap on. Microcook cheese mixture on 70% power for 3 to 5 minutes, stopping to stir well twice during cooking; stop cooking when the cheese is completely melted. Remove plastic wrap from edge of vegetable platter, drain liquid, then remove all wrap. Place serving utensils on the vegetables and in the cheese dip, gather around the coffee table, and allow your diners to serve themselves.

227 calories, 3 gm. fat, 15 gm. protein, 35 gm. carbohydrate, 10 mg. cholesterol, 126 mg. sodium, 5.2 gm. dietary fiber, 1317 RE vitamin A, 200 mg. vitamin C, 0 vitamin E as alpha tocopherol

Food exchange
1 skim milk, 1 bread/starch, 2 vegetable

Preparation time
20 minutes

Microcooking time
10 minutes

GARBANZO AND GREEN ONION DIP

8 servings, 1/3 cup each

15 oz. garbanzo beans, well-drained
1 Tbsp. vegetable oil
2 Tbsp. water
3 Tbsp. cider vinegar
1/2 cup finely chopped green onions
Garnish: 2 Tbsp. minced fresh parsley

Puree beans, oil, water, and vinegar in a blender. Blend until mixture is the consistency of a smooth paste. Transfer to a small mixing bowl; blend in chopped green onions. Garnish with fresh parsley. Serve with reduced-fat crackers such as Harvest Crisps or Reduced Fat Wheat Thins®.

106 calories, 4 gm. fat, 4 gm. protein, 14 gm. carbohydrate,
0 cholesterol, 14 mg. sodium, 6.2 gm. dietary fiber, 24 RE vitamin A,
8 mg. vitamin C, 0.8 mg. vitamin E as alpha tocopherol
(using sunflower oil)

Food exchange
1 bread/starch, 1/2 fat

Preparation time
10 minutes

GUACAMOLE MASQUERADE

8 servings, 1/8 cup each

10 oz. frozen green peas
1 jalapeno pepper, seeded and chopped into
small pieces
1 Tbsp. vegetable oil
2 tsp. lime juice
1/4 tsp. cumin
1/2 tsp. salt
Garnish: finely minced red onion

Place peas in a microwave-safe dish. Cover and microcook
on high power for 6 minutes. Drain well. Place cooked peas,
chopped pepper, and oil in a blender and process until
smooth. Turn into serving dish. Add lime juice, cumin and
salt just prior to serving with reduced-fat tortilla chips.
Garnish with minced red onion.

45 calories, 0 fat, 3 gm. protein, 6 gm. carbohydrate, 0 cholesterol,
267 mg. sodium, 1.1 gm. dietary fiber, 38 RE vitamin A,
7 mg. vitamin C, 0.8 mg. vitamin E as alpha tocopherol
(using sunflower oil)

Food exchange
2 vegetable

Preparation time
15 minutes

Microcooking time
6 minutes

LEMON FRUIT DIP

8 servings, 1/3 cup each

3-oz. pkg. nonfat cream cheese, softened
7 oz. marshmallow creme
2 tsp. finely grated lemon peel

Combine ingredients in a small mixing bowl. Microcook on 70% power for 2 minutes, stirring twice during cooking. Refrigerate until serving. This is tasty with whole strawberries, chunks of pineapple, and apple and pear slices.

88 calories, 0 fat, 0 protein, 21 gm. carbohydrate, 0 cholesterol, 31 mg. sodium, 0 dietary fiber, 13 RE vitamin A, 0 vitamin C, 0 vitamin E as alpha tocopherol

Food exchange
1 1/2 fruit

Preparation time
10 minutes

Microcooking time
2 minutes

MEXISKINS

8 servings, 1/2 potato each

4 large potatoes
1 Tbsp. vegetable oil
2 oz. reduced-fat Monterey Jack cheese, shredded
1/2 cup chunky-style mild salsa
1/2 cup nonfat sour cream
Garnish: parsley or chopped green onion top

Rub potatoes with oil. Microwave for 12 to 14 minutes, testing with a fork for doneness. Cut each potato in half. Scrape out the inside, leaving 1/4 inch of potato attached to the skin. Mix potato pulp with cheese, salsa, and sour cream. Stuff each potato skin with potato and cheese filling. Garnish with parsley or green onion tops. Broil for 4 to 6 minutes and serve.

150 calories, 1 gm. fat, 6 gm. protein, 29 gm. carbohydrate, 5 mg. cholesterol, 267 mg. sodium, 1.4 gm. dietary fiber, 56 RE vitamin A, 13 mg. vitamin C, 0.8 mg. vitamin E as alpha tocopherol (using sunflower oil)

Food exchange
2 bread/starch

Preparation time
15 minutes

Microcooking time
14 minutes

Broiling time
6 minutes

POLYNESIAN PEAR APPETIZER

8 servings, 1/2 pear each

3 oz. nonfat cream cheese, softened
1 Tbsp. powdered sugar
1/4 tsp. curry powder
1/4 cup flaked coconut
2 Tbsp. chopped pecans
4 ripe pears
2 Tbsp. lemon juice

Combine first five ingredients in a small mixing bowl. Cut pears in half. Remove the stem and core. Brush cut surfaces of pears with lemon juice to prevent browning. Stuff the center of the pears with cheese mixture. Serve immediately or chill up to 4 hours and serve. Pears become soft and loose color after 4 hours.

99 calories, 3 gm. fat, 1 gm. protein, 16 gm. carbohydrate,
0 cholesterol, 21 mg. sodium, 1.4 gm. dietary fiber, 15 RE vitamin A,
4 mg. vitamin C, 0.4 mg. vitamin E as alpha tocopherol

Food exchange
1 fruit, 1 fat

Preparation time
15 minutes

RANCH DIP FOR VEGGIES

12 servings, 1/4 cup each

1 large red bell pepper, chopped fine
1 large green onion, chopped fine
1 1-oz. pkg. buttermilk salad dressing mix
2 cups nonfat cottage cheese
Garnish: cherry tomato halves

Chop pepper and onion and set aside. In a blender, combine
salad dressing mix with cottage cheese. Blend until smooth.
Fold in raw peppers and onions. Transfer to a serving bowl
and garnish with cherry tomato halves. Serve with assorted
fresh vegetable dippers and reduced-fat party crackers.

32 calories, 0 fat, 6 gm. protein, 3 gm. carbohydrate, 0 cholesterol,
402 mg. sodium (to decrease sodium use 1/2 package dressing mix),
0 dietary fiber, 21 RE vitamin A, 0 vitamin C,
0 vitamin E as alpha tocopherol

Food exchange
1/2 lean meat

Preparation time
15 minutes

STUFFED MUSHROOMS

8 servings, 3 mushrooms each

1 lb. fresh mushrooms
1 carrot, finely grated
3 oz. nonfat cream cheese
2 Tbsp. fresh chives or 1 tsp. dried chives
1 Tbsp. grated fresh onion or 1 tsp.
minced dried onion

Wipe off mushroom caps. Remove stems and reserve for use as a topping on a pizza or in a fresh salad. Combine carrots, cream cheese, chives, and onion. Stuff into mushroom caps. Broil for 8 minutes. Serve hot.

27 calories, 0 fat, 2 gm. protein, 4 gm. carbohydrate, 0 cholesterol, 279 mg. sodium, 0.4 gm. dietary fiber, 267 RE vitamin A, 2 mg. vitamin C, 0 vitamin E as alpha tocopherol

Food exchange
1 vegetable

Preparation time
15 minutes

Broiling time
8 minutes

VEGETABLE PIZZA SQUARES

24 servings, 1/24 of 15-inch by 8-inch jelly roll pan

1 8-roll tube of crescent dinner rolls
3 oz. nonfat cream cheese, softened
1/2 cup reduced-fat ranch-style buttermilk salad
  dressing
4 cups assorted raw vegetables, cut in 1/2-inch
  pieces (try cauliflower, green and red pepper,
  carrots, broccoli)
Garnish: chopped fresh chives

Preheat oven to 375° F. Remove rolls from the tube and
press flat into a 15-inch by 8-inch jelly roll pan that has
been sprayed with non-stick cooking spray. Pat out to form
a crust. Bake for 8 to 10 minutes until lightly browned.
Cool crust for 20 minutes. Meanwhile, combine softened
cream cheese with salad dressing; spread over cooled crust.
Spread chopped vegetables over dressing and garnish with
chives. Refrigerate until serving.

52 calories, 2 gm. fat, 1 gm. protein, 7 gm. carbohydrate,
1 mg. cholesterol, 166 mg. sodium, 0.2 gm. dietary fiber,
233 RE vitamin A, 18 mg. vitamin C, 0 vitamin E as alpha tocopherol

Food exchange
1 vegetable, 1/2 bread/starch

Preparation time
15 minutes

Baking time
10 minutes

Cooling time
20 minutes

BEVERAGES

CREAMY PAPAYA COOLER

8 servings, 3/4 cup each

2 papaya, peeled, seeded, and cubed
6-oz. can frozen limeade concentrate
1 cup water
1 cup nonfat lemon yogurt
Garnish: twisted slices of fresh lime

Combine all ingredients in a blender and process until smooth. Serve in short glasses, garnished with a twisted slice of lime.

83 calories, 0 fat, 2 gm. protein, 20 gm. carbohydrate, 0 cholesterol, 26 mg. sodium, 1.4 gm. dietary fiber, 153 RE vitamin A, 49 mg. vitamin C, 0 vitamin E as alpha tocopherol

Food exchange
1 1/2 fruit

Preparation time
15 minutes

FRESH TOMATO COCKTAIL

8 servings, 6 oz. each

4 large ripe tomatoes
1 small green pepper
1 small onion
1 stalk celery
1 Tbsp. sugar
1/2 tsp. black pepper
1/4 tsp. Tabasco®, optional
Garnish: celery leaves

In a food processor or blender, combine quartered tomatoes with pepper, onion, and celery in two batches. Puree until smooth. Transfer to a large serving pitcher. Stir in sugar and pepper and optional Tabasco. Serve chilled with celery leaves as a garnish.

29 calories, 0 fat, 0 protein, 6 gm. carbohydrate, 0 cholesterol, 10 mg. sodium, 0.8 gm. dietary fiber, 57 RE vitamin A, 37 mg. vitamin C, 0 vitamin E as alpha tocopherol

Food exchange
1 vegetable

Preparation time
15 minutes

HAWAIIAN FRUIT DRINK

10 servings, 8 oz. each

46 oz. cranberry-raspberry juice
12 oz. frozen lemonade concentrate
12 oz. water
12 oz. sugar-free lemon-lime soft drink
Garnish: pineapple chunks

Mix first three ingredients in a punch bowl or large pitcher. Just before serving, add soft drink. Serve over crushed ice. Garnish with pineapple chunks on a skewer.

132 calories, 0 fat, 0 protein, 33 gm. carbohydrate, 0 cholesterol,
8 mg. sodium, 0 dietary fiber, 3 RE vitamin A, 47 mg. vitamin C,
0 vitamin E as alpha tocopherol

Food exchange
2 fruit

Preparation time
10 minutes

HOLIDAY TEA

10 servings, 8 oz. each

1 cup water
1/4 cup sugar (optional)
1 stick cinnamon
1 tsp. ground cloves
46 oz. cranberry juice
1 quart orange juice
1/4 cup lemon juice

In a small saucepan, combine water, sugar, cinnamon, and cloves. Boil for 15 minutes. Remove cinnamon stick. To serve cold, combine spiced syrup with cranberry, orange, and lemon juice in a punch bowl. Garnish bowl with an ice mold made with sprigs of holly. To serve hot, combine spiced syrup with cranberry, orange, and lemon juice in a percolator. Remove basket and tubing. Heat through, and garnish each mug with a cinnamon stick.

145 calories (120 calories without sugar), 0 fat, 0 protein, 36 gm. carbohydrate (30 gm. carbohydrate without sugar), 0 cholesterol, 12 mg. sodium, 0 dietary fiber, 5 RE vitamin A, 93 mg. vitamin C, 0 vitamin E as alpha tocopherol

Food exchange
2 1/2 fruit (2 fruit without sugar)

Preparation time
10 minutes

Cooking time
15 minutes

Heating time for percolator punch
25 minutes

KARLA'S ROSY PUNCH

Thanks to Karla Palmer for this quick and delicious summer-time party drink.

20 servings, 6 oz. each

1 46-oz. can pineapple juice
1 46-oz. bottle reduced-calorie cranberry juice
 cocktail
1 Tbsp. almond extract
2 quarts sugar-free lemon-lime soft drink

Mix juices with almond extract and chill. Add soft drink just before serving.

54 calories, 0 fat, 1 gm. protein, 13 gm. carbohydrate, 0 cholesterol, 3 mg. sodium, 0 dietary fiber, 1 RE vitamin A, 30 mg. vitamin C, 0 vitamin E as alpha tocopherol

Food exchange
1 fruit

Preparation time
10 minutes

SEAFOAM PUNCH

14 servings, 8 oz. each

1 package sugar-free lemon-lime soft drink powder
2 cups skim milk
46 oz. pineapple juice
2 cups lime sherbet
12 oz. sugar-free lemon-lime soft drink
Garnish: fresh mint or finely chopped
     wintergreen candy

Mix soft drink powder with milk in a punch bowl or large pitcher. Add pineapple juice. Just before serving, add sherbet and chilled sugar-free lemon lime drink.

Garnish cups with a sprig of fresh mint or sprinkles of finely chopped wintergreen candy.

117 calories, 0 fat, 1 gm. protein, 26 gm. carbohydrate,
2 mg. cholesterol, 30 mg. sodium, 0 dietary fiber, 21 RE vitamin A,
11 mg. vitamin C, 0 vitamin E as alpha tocopherol

Food exchange
2 fruit

Preparation time
10 minutes

SNAP OUT OF IT!

4 servings, 8 oz. each

1 Tbsp. lime juice
1 quart vegetable juice cocktail
2 tsp. Worcestershire sauce
Dash ground pepper
Dash Tabasco® sauce
Ice cubes
Garnish: slice of lemon and a stalk of celery

Combine first five ingredients in a glass pitcher. Serve over ice. Garnish glasses with lemon slices and celery stalks.

43 calories, 0 fat, 1 gm. protein, 10 gm. carbohydrate, 0 cholesterol, 826 mg. sodium, 1.4 gm. dietary fiber, 265 RE vitamin A, 62 mg. vitamin C, 0 vitamin E as alpha tocopherol

Food exchange
2 vegetable

Preparation time
10 minutes

SPARKLING PUNCH

16 servings, 8 oz. each

2 qt. apple cider
6 oz. frozen grape juice concentrate
3 cups water
1 qt. gingerale
Garnish: ice ring with flowers

Mix the ingredients together in a punch bowl just before serving. Garnish with a molded ice ring of plastic flowers.

107 calories, 0 fat, 0 protein, 26 gm. carbohydrate, 0 cholesterol, 8 mg. sodium, 0 dietary fiber, 8 RE vitamin A, 15 mg. vitamin C, 0 vitamin E as alpha tocopherol

Food exchange
2 fruit

Preparation time
10 minutes

SPICED CIDER

Who needs potpourri when you've got cider steeping!

10 servings, 6 oz. each

2 cups cranberry juice
1 1/2 qt. apple cider
1/4 cup brown sugar (optional)
2 broken cinnamon sticks
2 tsp. grated orange peel
6 whole cloves

Mix first three ingredients in a 12-cup percolator.
Combine cinnamon sticks, orange peel, and cloves in the
top basket. Percolate and serve hot.

119 calories (100 calories without brown sugar), 0 fat, 0 protein,
30 gm. carbohydrate, 0 cholesterol, 8 mg. sodium, 0 dietary fiber,
0 vitamin A, 22 mg. vitamin C, 0 vitamin E as alpha tocopherol

Food exchange
2 fruit (1 1/2 fruit without brown sugar)

Preparation time
10 minutes

Percolating time
15 minutes

STRAWBERRY DAIQUIRI

4 servings, 6 oz. each

2 cups fresh strawberries
1/4 cup frozen limeade concentrate
1 cup crushed ice
2 tsp. rum extract
Garnish: fresh strawberries

Combine all ingredients in a blender until smooth.

Serve in short beverage glasses with a fresh strawberry garnish.

48 calories, 0 fat, 0 protein, 12 gm. carbohydrate, 0 cholesterol,
2 mg. sodium, 0 dietary fiber, 2 RE vitamin A, 42 mg. vitamin C,
0 vitamin E as alpha tocopherol

Food exchange
1 fruit

Preparation time
15 minutes

STRAWBERRY ICED TEA

8 servings, 8 oz. each

1 cup orange juice
1/4 cup sugar (or equivalent sugar substitute)
1/3 cup instant tea
10 oz. frozen strawberries, thawed
4 cups water
2 cups crushed ice
Garnish: fresh lemon wedges

Combine first four ingredients in a blender and blend until smooth. Pour into a 2-quart pitcher and add water and ice. Serve in iced tea glasses with a fresh lemon-wedge garnish.

81 calories (55 with sugar substitute), 0 fat, 0 protein,
20 gm. carbohydrate, 0 cholesterol, 2 mg. sodium, 0 dietary fiber,
2 RE vitamin A, 18 mg. vitamin C, 0 vitamin E as alpha tocopherol

Food exchange
1 1/2 fruit (1 fruit with sugar substitute)

Preparation time
10 minutes

SUMMER SLUSH

16 servings, 8 oz. each

6 oz. frozen orange juice concentrate
6 oz. pink lemonade concentrate
46 oz. pineapple juice
46 oz. apricot nectar
36 oz. (3 12-oz. cans) sugar-free lemon-lime
   soft drink
Garnish: melon balls on swizzle sticks

Combine first four ingredients in a large plastic container and freeze. One hour before serving, remove from the freezer. Use a heavy, long-handled metal spoon to break up slush for serving. Scoop 6 ounces slush into a short glass and pour in 2 ounces of soft drink. Garnish each glass with a melon ball on a swizzle stick.

140 calories, 0 fat, 0 protein, 35 gm. carbohydrate, 0 cholesterol, 6 mg. sodium, 0 dietary fiber, 125 RE vitamin A, 30 mg. vitamin C, 0 vitamin E as alpha tocopherol

Food exchange
2 fruit

Preparation time
10 minutes

SOUPS

ANY VEGETABLE BROTH-BASED SOUP

8 servings, 1 cup each

1 20-oz. pkg. frozen vegetables of choice
46 oz. canned tomato juice or 1 1/2 qt. water
3 oz. ramen noodles with beef or chicken flavoring
2 tsp. oregano, parsley, or herb of choice

Suggested combinations:

1. Mixed vegetables, tomato juice, beef-flavored ramen, oregano
2. Stew vegetables, water, beef-flavored ramen, parsley
3. California blend vegetables, water, chicken-flavored ramen, parsley
4. Stir-fry blend vegetables, water, chicken-flavored ramen, parsley

Mix vegetables and tomato juice or water in a 5-qt. pan. Heat to boiling. Add noodles, flavor packet, and herb of choice. Simmer for 15 minutes, stirring often.

151 calories, 0 fat, 6 gm. protein, 30 gm. carbohydrate, 0 cholesterol, 750 mg. sodium, 2.2 gm. dietary fiber, 393 RE vitamin A, 32 mg. vitamin C, 0 vitamin E as alpha tocopherol

Food exchange
2 vegetable, 1 bread/starch

Preparation time
10 minutes

Cooking time
15 minutes

ANY VEGETABLE CREAM SOUP

8 servings, 1 cup each

4 cups diced raw vegetables (try a combination of
potatoes, carrots, celery, onion, broccoli,
Brussels sprouts, cauliflower, asparagus)
1 cup water
1 chicken bouillon cube
1 13-oz. can reduced-fat cream of chicken soup
1 1/2 cups skim milk
4 oz. reduced-fat American processed cheese,
cubed
Garnish: crunchy bread sticks

Combine vegetables, water, and bouillon cube in a stockpot. Bring to a boil, and then reduce heat; simmer for 20
minutes. Add chicken soup and milk. Bring to a boil and
stir in cheese. Serve when cheese is melted. Garnish with
crunchy breadsticks.

122 calories, 4 gm. fat, 8 gm. protein, 17 gm. carbohydrate,
4 mg. cholesterol, 769 mg. sodium (to decrease sodium, use
reduced-sodium bouillon), 1.6 gm. dietary fiber, 894 RE vitamin A,
35 mg. vitamin C, 0 vitamin E as alpha tocopherol

Food exchange
1 bread/starch, 2 vegetable

Preparation time
15 minutes

Cooking time
20 minutes

CHILLED TOMATO SOUP

8 servings, 1 cup each

1 Tbsp. vegetable oil
1 lb. carrots, scrubbed well and thinly sliced
1 large onion, chopped fine
1/4 tsp. garlic powder
8 medium fresh tomatoes, peeled and chopped
14-oz. can no-added-salt chicken broth
1/2 tsp. basil
1/2 tsp. thyme
1/2 tsp. salt
1/4 tsp. white pepper
1 cup evaporated skim milk
1 tsp. sugar

In a large stockpot, heat oil over medium heat. Add sliced carrots, onion, and garlic powder; cook for 5 minutes. Add tomatoes, broth, basil, thyme, salt, and pepper and heat through, about 5 minutes, over medium heat. Remove from heat and stir in skim milk and sugar. Chill mixture for at least 2 hours. Ladle into bowls and garnish with a sprinkle of Parmesan cheese.

88 calories, 2 gm. fat, 2 gm. protein, 15 gm. carbohydrate,
0 cholesterol, 180 mg. sodium, 2.5 gm. dietary fiber, 1688 RE vitamin A, 30 mg. vitamin C, 0.8 mg. vitamin E as alpha tocopherol
(using sunflower oil)

Food exchange
2 vegetable, 1/2 skim milk

Preparation time
20 minutes

Chilling time
2 hours

CHILLED VEGETABLE SOUP

8 servings, 1 cup each

4 large carrots, coarsely chopped
14-oz. can chunky tomatoes or 2 large tomatoes,
    peeled and chopped
1 large cucumber, peeled, seeded, and chopped
2 medium green peppers, seeded and chopped
1 medium zucchini, shredded
2 large ribs celery, chopped fine
1 large red onion, chopped fine
2 cloves garlic, minced
3 cups no-added-salt tomato juice
2 Tbsp. vegetable oil
1/4 cup cider vinegar
1 tsp. salt
1 Tbsp. lemon juice
1/2 tsp. Tabasco® sauce
1 tsp. oregano
1/2 tsp. fennel

Stir together all ingredients, cover, and refrigerate at least
2 hours. Garnish with croutons.

95 calories, 3 gm. fat, 2 gm. protein, 15 gm. carbohydrate, 0 cholesterol, 412 mg. sodium, 2.6 gm. dietary fiber, 1144 RE vitamin A,
82 mg. vitamin C, 0 vitamin E as alpha tocopherol

Food exchange
3 vegetable, 1/2 fat

Preparation time
25 minutes

Chilling time
2 hours

CREAM OF ASPARAGUS SOUP

8 servings, 1 cup each

2 lb. clean tender asparagus, chopped in 1/4-inch
    slices
3 scallions, chopped fine
1 Tbsp. vegetable oil
1 cup nonfat cottage cheese
1 cup evaporated skim milk
46-oz. can no-added-salt chicken broth
1/4 tsp. curry powder
1/4 tsp. white pepper
1 tsp. dill weed

In a large stockpot, heat oil and saute chopped asparagus
and green onion for 6 to 8 minutes. Put half of the cooked
onion and asparagus into a blender with the cottage cheese
and milk. Process until smooth. Add broth to the stockpot
and stir to mix. Using a whisk, gradually add vegetable and
milk mixture to the broth and vegetables. Heat just to
scalding, stirring continually to prevent scorching. Reduce
heat immediately. Stir in seasonings and serve.

86 calories, 2 gm. fat, 9 gm. protein, 9 gm. carbohydrate, 3 mg.
cholesterol, 134 mg. sodium, 1 gm. dietary fiber, 144 RE vitamin A,
37 mg. vitamin C, 1.3 mg. vitamin E as alpha tocopherol
(using sunflower oil)

Food exchange
1/2 skim milk, 1 vegetable, 1/2 fat

Preparation time
15 minutes

Cooking time
15 minutes

FRENCH ONION SOUP

8 servings, 1 cup each

6 medium yellow onions, thinly sliced
2 Tbsp. margarine
1 qt. (32 oz.) beef broth
1 Tbsp. Worcestershire sauce
1/8 tsp. pepper
8 slices French bread
2 oz. part-skim mozzarella cheese, shredded

In a large saucepan, cook sliced onions in margarine until tender, about 15 minutes. Add beef broth, Worcestershire sauce, and pepper. Bring to a boil. Meanwhile, sprinkle French bread with shredded cheese and place under the broiler for 3 minutes. Ladle soup into bowls, and garnish with slices of bread.

225 calories, 4 gm. fat, 8 gm. protein, 37 gm. carbohydrate, 4 mg. cholesterol, 1005 mg. sodium (to decrease sodium, choose reduced-sodium broth), 1.8 gm. dietary fiber, 37 RE vitamin A, 8 mg. vitamin C, 0.8 mg. vitamin E as alpha tocopherol (using soft Mazola ®)

Food exchange
1 1/2 bread/starch, 1 fat, 2 vegetable

Preparation time
20 minutes

GARDEN TOMATO SOUP WITH CREAM

8 servings, 1 cup each

1 tsp. margarine
1 scallion, chopped fine
2 Tbsp. chopped fresh parsley
6 large ripe tomatoes, peeled and cut into chunks
1 qt. no-added-salt chicken broth
3 Tbsp. flour
14-oz. can evaporated skim milk
1 cup nonfat sour cream
1/2 tsp. salt
1/4 tsp. white pepper

In a large stockpot, saute scallion and parsley in margarine. Add tomato chunks and chicken broth and cook over medium heat for 5 minutes. Lower heat to simmer. In a shaker container, mix flour with skim milk until smooth. Using a whisk, blend this mixture into the tomatoes, stirring constantly. Bring mixture to a boil, then immediately reduce heat again to simmer. Use a ladle to remove 1/2 cup of tomato mixture and combine it with sour cream in a small bowl. Blend until smooth and then return this to soup. Heat through. Add salt and pepper. Serve with reduced-fat string cheese and wheat crackers.

119 calories, 3 gm. fat, 7 gm. protein, 17 gm. carbohydrate, 1 mg. cholesterol, 247 mg. sodium, 0 dietary fiber, 292 RE vitamin A, 23 mg. vitamin C, 0 vitamin E as alpha tocopherol

Food exchange
1 skim milk, 1 vegetable

Preparation time
15 minutes

Cooking time
20 minutes

GAZPACHO

8 servings, 3/4 cup each

3 cloves fresh garlic, minced
3 Tbsp. white vinegar
1/2 tsp. salt
1 tsp. vegetable oil
1 tsp. tarragon
1 tsp. sugar
1 24-oz. can vegetable juice cocktail, divided
1 large green pepper, halved and seeded
1 large cucumber, pared
2 ribs of celery
2 medium tomatoes, peeled and quartered

In a large bowl, combine minced garlic, vinegar, salt, oil, tarragon, sugar, and 2 cups of vegetable juice cocktail. In a blender or food processor, process pepper, cucumber, celery, and tomatoes, with 1 cup of the vegetable juice cocktail until finely chopped. Add to garlic and vinegar mixture. Chill at least 30 minutes. Ladle into bowls and serve as a first course to a summer dinner. Garnish with long thin breadsticks, or enjoy with reduced-fat cheese and crackers for a lunch treat.

44 calories, 0 fat, 1 gm. protein, 9 gm. carbohydrate, 0 cholesterol, 424 mg. sodium, 0.6 gm. dietary fiber, 270 RE vitamin A, 48 mg. vitamin C, 0 vitamin E as alpha tocopherol

Food exchange
2 vegetable

Preparation time
15 minutes

Chilling time
30 minutes

HAM AND BEAN SOUP

8 servings, 1 cup each

2 cups dry navy or pinto beans
2 qt. water
4 oz. lean ham, shredded
1 small onion, diced
1 tsp. salt
1 bay leaf
3 Tbsp. Worcestershire sauce
3 large carrots, scrubbed and sliced thin

In a large stockpot, combine all ingredients except the carrots, and bring to a boil. Reduce heat to a simmer; cover
and cook for 2 1/2 hours or until beans are tender. Add the
carrots 30 minutes before the end of the cooking time to
ensure a favorable texture. Remove the bay leaf, then serve
with corn bread muffins.

201 calories, 1 gm. fat, 13 gm. protein, 34 gm. carbohydrate,
7 mg. cholesterol, 476 mg. sodium, 3.4 gm. dietary fiber, 759 RE
vitamin A, 9 mg. vitamin C, 0 vitamin E as alpha tocopherol

Food exchange
1 lean meat, 1 1/2 bread/starch, 1 vegetable

Preparation time
15 minutes

Cooking time
2 1/2 hours

ITALIAN HARVEST SOUP

8 servings, 1 cup each

1/4 lb. reduced-fat spicy sausage
1 large onion, sliced
2 carrots, chopped
1 Tbsp. vegetable oil
3 14-oz. cans no-added-salt beef broth
1 16-oz. can diced tomatoes with juice
1/8 tsp. cayenne pepper
1/4 tsp. salt
1/2 tsp. oregano
1/2 tsp. marjoram
1 bay leaf
1/2 tsp. summer savory
10 oz. frozen green beans
8 oz. fresh mushrooms, sliced
1/4 head cabbage, shredded
Garnish: cubes of French bread and shredded part-
skim mozzarella cheese

In a large stockpot, brown sausage with onion and carrots.
Drain well. Add all remaining ingredients and bring to a
boil. Reduce to a simmer and continue cooking for 20
minutes. Remove bay leaf, and ladle soup into bowls.
Garnish with cubes of French bread and shredded part-
skim mozzarella cheese.

122 calories, 6 gm. fat, 5 gm. protein, 12 gm. carbohydrate,
11 mg. cholesterol, 406 mg. sodium, 2.4 gm. dietary fiber,
83 RE vitamin A, 25 mg. vitamin C, 0.9 mg. vitamin E as
alpha tocopherol (using sunflower oil)

Food exchange
2 vegetable, 1/2 lean meat, 1 fat

Preparation time
20 minutes

Cooking time
25 minutes

LENTIL CARROT SOUP

8 servings, 1 cup each

1 lb. dry lentils
2 1/2 qt. water
8 slices bacon, diced fine
3 large carrots, diced
1 large onion, diced
2 ribs celery, cut fine
1 bay leaf
1/8 tsp. thyme
1/2 tsp. salt
1/4 tsp. black pepper
2 Tbsp. fresh parsley, minced

Combine lentils and water in a large pot. Bring to a boil and then reduce heat. Cover and simmer for 45 minutes. Meanwhile, cook bacon until crisp and drain well. Add crisped bacon, vegetables, and spices to the lentils. Simmer for 20 minutes, and serve.

228 calories, 4 gm. fat, 16 gm. protein, 33 gm. carbohydrate, 6 mg. cholesterol, 272 mg. sodium, 6.6 gm. dietary fiber, 781 RE vitamin A, 15 mg. vitamin C, 0 vitamin E as alpha tocopherol

Food exchange
1 lean meat, 1 vegetable, 2 bread/starch

Preparation time
15 minutes

Cooking time
1 hour, 5 minutes

PEANUT LOVER'S BEAN SOUP

8 servings, 1 cup each

1 tsp. margarine
3 large carrots, scrubbed and sliced thin
1 large white onion, diced
1 large green pepper, diced
4 oz. lean roast beef, shredded
2 cups no-added-salt beef broth
1 16-oz. can black-eyed peas, drained
1 16-oz. can pinto or navy beans, drained
1 tsp. salt
1/8 tsp. cayenne pepper
1/2 cup salted peanuts, chopped
1 Tbsp. basil
1 tsp. ground coriander

In a large stockpot, saute carrots, onions, and peppers in margarine for 5 minutes. Add all remaining ingredients. Bring to a boil, then reduce to a simmer. Cook uncovered for 20 minutes, and serve with a green salad and corn bread.

257 calories, 9 gm. fat, 15 gm. protein, 34 gm. carbohydrate, 11 mg. cholesterol, 947 mg. sodium (to decrease sodium, use unsalted peanuts), 7.4 gm. dietary fiber, 783 RE vitamin A, 28 mg. vitamin C, 0 vitamin E as alpha tocopherol

Food exchange
1 fat, 1 lean meat, 1 vegetable, 1 1/2 bread/starch

Preparation time
15 minutes

Cooking time
25 minutes

SPICY BEEF AND BLACK BEAN SOUP

8 servings, 1 cup each

1 lb. black beans
3 qt. water
4 oz. lean roast beef, shredded
1 large carrot, scrubbed and sliced
1 large white onion, chopped fine
4 whole cloves
1/8 tsp. red pepper
1/2 cup sherry
1 Tbsp. lemon juice
Garnish: chopped, hard-boiled egg whites

Place first seven ingredients in a large stockpot. Bring mixture to a boil. Reduce heat, cover, and cook slowly for 2 1/2 hours or until beans are very soft. Remove half of the mixture to a blender and process until almost smooth. Return the pureed portion to the stockpot, stir in sherry and lemon juice and serve. Garnish with chopped egg whites, if desired.

113 calories, 1 gm. fat, 8 gm. protein, 13 gm. carbohydrate, 11 mg. cholesterol, 295 mg. sodium, 3.8 gm. dietary fiber, 253 RE vitamin A, 3 mg. vitamin C, 0 vitamin E as alpha tocopherol

Food exchange
1 lean meat, 1 bread/starch

Preparation time
10 minutes

Cooking time
2 1/2 hours

SUMMER SQUASH SOUP

8 servings, 1 cup each

2 14-oz. cans beef broth
3 medium yellow squash, sliced thin
1 large white onion, diced
1/4 tsp. black pepper
1/2 cup plain yogurt

In a large stockpot, combine broth, sliced squash, onion, and pepper. Bring to a boil, then reduce heat and simmer for 10 minutes. Pour mixture into a blender and process until nearly smooth. Fold in yogurt and serve.

52 calories, 0 fat, 3 gm. protein, 9 gm. carbohydrate, 1 mg. cholesterol, 569 mg. sodium, 0 dietary fiber, 29 RE vitamin A, 20 mg. vitamin C, 0 vitamin E as alpha tocopherol

Food exchange
2 vegetable

Preparation time
10 minutes

Cooking time
15 minutes

SWEET POTATO SOUP

8 servings, 1 cup each

1 tsp. margarine
1 large onion, chopped
3 ribs celery, diced
2 cups chicken broth
5 sweet potatoes, peeled and cut into chunks
3 large carrots, sliced thin
1 tsp. salt
1/4 tsp. garlic powder
1/4 tsp. white pepper
2 cups skim milk

Melt margarine in a stockpot. Add onion and celery, and cook for 10 minutes. Add broth, sweet potatoes, carrots, salt, garlic powder, and white pepper, and bring to a boil. Simmer for 20 minutes or until sweet potatoes are tender. Puree soup or use a masher and break up the sweet potatoes to desired consistency. Stir in milk and warm through. Serve with a cold roast beef sandwich.

123 calories, 0 fat, 4 gm. protein, 25 gm. carbohydrate, 1 mg. cholesterol, 334 mg. sodium, 6.5 gm. dietary fiber, 2359 RE vitamin A, 23 mg. vitamin C, 3.7 mg. vitamin E as alpha tocopherol

Food exchange
1 bread/starch, 2 vegetable

Preparation time
10 minutes

Cooking time
30 minutes

SWISS ONION SOUP

The creamy cousin to the more famous French variety.

8 servings, 1 cup each

6 large onions, finely chopped
2 Tbsp. margarine
4 cups evaporated skim milk
2 cups water
4 oz. reduced-fat Swiss cheese, grated
1/2 tsp. salt
1/4 tsp. white pepper
1/2 tsp. paprika
Garnish: 1/2 cup croutons

In a stockpot, cook onions in margarine until soft but still white. Do not brown. Stir in milk and water, and bring to a slow boil. Add grated cheese, salt, pepper, and paprika. Simmer, covered, over low heat for 10 minutes, stirring occasionally. Ladle into soup bowls, and garnish with croutons.

230 calories, 5 gm. fat, 15 gm. protein, 29 gm. carbohydrate, 13 mg. cholesterol, 340 mg. sodium, 2.6 gm. dietary fiber, 186 RE vitamin A, 12 mg. vitamin C, 0.8 mg. vitamin E as alpha tocopherol (using soft Mazola®)

Food exchange
1 fat, 1 skim milk, 2 vegetable, 1/2 bread/starch

Preparation time
10 minutes

Cooking time
20 minutes

TURNIP AND MIXED VEGETABLE SOUP WITH BARLEY

8 servings, 1 cup each

1 46-oz. can no-added-salt beef broth
1 16-oz. can chopped tomatoes with juice
2/3 cup pearl barley
2 large carrots, scrubbed and sliced thin
2 white turnips, scrubbed, peeled, and chopped
1 large white onion, chopped
1 small green pepper, diced
1 bay leaf
1 tsp. sugar

Combine all ingredients in a stockpot and bring to a boil. Reduce heat to a simmer and cook uncovered for 20 minutes. Remove bay leaf. Serve with breadsticks, cottage cheese, and fruit salad.

58 calories, 0 fat, 1 gm. protein, 13 gm. carbohydrate, 0 cholesterol, 163 mg. sodium, 5.2 gm. dietary fiber, 548 RE vitamin A, 22 mg. vitamin C, 0 vitamin E as alpha tocopherol

Food exchange
1 vegetable, 1/2 bread/starch

Preparation time
15 minutes

Cooking time
25 minutes

FRUIT SOUPS

BLUEBERRY BISQUE

4 servings, 1 cup each

1 1/2 cups apple juice
1/2 cup evaporated skim milk
1 cup nonfat sour cream
2 tsp. sugar-free cherry drink powder
(such as Kool-Aid®)
2 cup fresh blueberries, washed and sorted

In a large bowl, use a whisk to combine apple juice with skim milk; continue, whisking the sour cream into the juice and milk. Stir in drink powder until fully dissolved. Fold in blueberries. Chill for at least 30 minutes. Serve.

93 calories, 0 fat, 1 gm. protein, 22 gm. carbohydrate, 0 cholesterol, 21 mg. sodium, 0 dietary fiber, 21 RE vitamin A, 10 mg. vitamin C, 0 vitamin E as alpha tocopherol

Food Exchange
1 1/2 fruit

Preparation time
10 minutes

Chilling time
30 minutes

HOT CHERRY COMPOTE

12 servings, 3/4 cup each

8 oz. dried prunes, pitted
8 oz. dried apricots
20 oz. pineapple chunks with juice
1/4 cup sherry
1 large can cherry pie filling

Preheat oven to 350° F. Place dried fruit in the bottom of a baking dish. Layer the pineapple and juice on top. Sprinkle with sherry. Spread the cherry pie filling on top. Bake uncovered for 30 minutes. To microcook: cook on high power for 12 to 15 minutes. Serve warm as a side dish with pork.

152 calories, 0 fat, 1 gm. protein, 38 gm. carbohydrate, 0 cholesterol, 6 mg. sodium, 1.2 gm. dietary fiber, 97 RE vitamin A, 6 mg. vitamin C, 0 vitamin E as alpha tocopherol

Food Exchange
2 1/2 fruit

Preparation time
10 minutes

Baking time
30 minutes

Microcooking time
15 minutes

ORANGE FRUIT SOUP

8 servings, 3/4 cup each

2 Tbsp. quick-cooking tapioca
2 1/2 cups orange juice
1 tsp. allspice
3 large ice cubes
1 11-oz. can mandarin oranges, drained well
2 ripe nectarines, peeled and cut into
   bite-sized pieces
Garnish: finely grated orange rind

In a small saucepan, combine tapioca, orange juice, and allspice. Bring to a boil over medium heat. Remove from heat and stir in 3 large ice cubes. When ice is melted, fold in drained oranges and nectarines. Garnish each bowl of soup with finely grated orange rind.

75 calories, 0 fat, 1 gm. protein, 18 gm. carbohydrate, 0 cholesterol, 2 mg. sodium, 0 dietary fiber, 46 RE vitamin A, 46 mg. vitamin C, 0 vitamin E as alpha tocopherol

Food Exchange
1 1/2 fruit

Preparation time
15 minutes

PEARS AND BERRIES SOUP

This recipe is a favorite of mine from the American Institute for Cancer Research Newsletter

8 servings, 3/4 cup each

6 pears, peeled, cored, and chopped
1 1/3 cups fresh or frozen raspberries (reserve 8 whole berries for garnish)
1/2 tsp. cinnamon
3 cups cranberry-raspberry beverage

Puree the pears, berries, and cinnamon in a blender or food processor. Add the cranberry-raspberry beverage, and blend again. Chill until serving time. Garnish each serving with a whole raspberry.

◆

138 calories, 0 fat, 0 protein, 34 gm. carbohydrate, 0 cholesterol, 2 mg. sodium, 3 gm. dietary fiber, 4 RE vitamin A, 10 mg. vitamin C, 0.6 mg. vitamin E as alpha tocopherol

Food exchange
2 1/2 fruit

Preparation time
15 minutes

RED GRAPE SOUP

8 servings, 3/4 cup each

1 1/2 cups water
1/4 cup sugar
1 stick cinnamon
2 cups red grape juice
3 Tbsp. quick-cooking tapioca
6 oz. frozen orange-pineapple juice concentrate
2 cups red seedless grapes, halved
1/2 cup red wine
Garnish: nonfat lemon yogurt

In a medium saucepan, combine water, sugar, cinnamon, and grape juice. Bring this to a boil and then add tapioca. Cook for 5 minutes, stirring occasionally. Remove from heat and add frozen juice concentrate, grapes, and wine. Chill until serving time. Garnish each bowl of fruit soup with a dollop of nonfat lemon yogurt.

131 calories, 0 fat, 0 protein, 31 gm. carbohydrate, 0 cholesterol, 2 mg. sodium, 0 dietary fiber, 75 RE vitamin A, 17 mg. vitamin C, 0 vitamin E as alpha tocopherol

Food Exchange
2 fruit

Preparation time
10 minutes

Cooking time
10 minutes

SWEDISH FRUIT SOUP

8 servings, 3/4 cup each

3/4 cup dried apricots
3/4 cup dried pineapple
1/2 cup dried pears
1/2 cup golden raisins
2 qt. water
1 cinnamon stick
1/3 cup grenadine
3 Tbsp. tapioca

Combine fruit and water in a stockpot. Add cinnamon, and cook over low heat for 15 minutes. Combine tapioca with grenadine in a small bowl. Whisk tapioca into the hot fruit mixture, bring to a boil, and stir until thick. Cover and refrigerate at least 2 hours before serving. The Swedes prefer this fruit soup garnished with real whipping cream!

114 calories, 0 fat, 1 gm. protein, 29 gm. carbohydrate, 0 cholesterol, 3 mg. sodium, 1.2 gm. dietary fiber, 1021 RE vitamin A, 5 mg. vitamin C, 0.3 mg. vitamin E as alpha tocopherol

Food exchange
2 fruit

Preparation time
10 minutes

Cooking time
20 minutes

Chilling time
2 hours

FRUIT SALADS

BESS'S PINEAPPLE SALAD

A favorite from the Ingleside Club.

12 servings, 1/2 cup each

20-oz. can crushed pineapple, not drained
6 oz. fat-free cream cheese, softened
3-oz. pkg. instant vanilla pudding (dry)
20-oz. can pineapple chunks, drained
8 oz. reduced-fat whipped topping
Garnish: fresh mint

Combine crushed pineapple and juice with softened cream cheese and pudding mix. Blend until smooth. Fold in drained pineapple chunks and whipped topping. Chill at least 2 hours before serving.

119 calories, 2 gm. fat, 2 gm. protein, 24 gm. carbohydrate, 0 cholesterol, 27 mg. sodium, 1.4 gm. dietary fiber, 127 RE vitamin A, 121 mg. vitamin C, 0 vitamin E as alpha tocopherol

Food exchange
2 fruit

Preparation time
15 minutes

Chilling time
2 hours

CHERRY AMBROSIA

8 servings, 3/4 cup each

2 cups fresh bing cherries, washed, pitted,
and chopped
1 cup seedless green grapes, washed and halved
3 fresh oranges, peeled, cut in half, sectioned,
and cut into bite-sized pieces
1/4 cup flaked coconut
3 oz. nonfat cream cheese
3 Tbsp. frozen orange juice concentrate

In a large salad bowl, combine cherries, grapes, oranges, and coconut. In a microwave-safe bowl, soften cream cheese by heating on high power for 45 seconds. Mix the orange juice concentrate with the cream cheese until no lumps remain. Pour over fruit mixture, and serve or refrigerate.

100 calories, 1 gm. fat, 2 gm. protein, 22 gm. carbohydrate,
0 cholesterol, 18 mg. sodium, 3.2 gm. dietary fiber, 34 RE vitamin A,
42 mg. vitamin C, 0 vitamin E as alpha tocopherol

Food exchange
1 1/2 fruit

Preparation time
15 minutes

CINNAMON ORANGE SALAD

8 servings, 3/4 cup each

6 oranges, peeled and cut into bite-size pieces
1 cup miniature marshmallows
1 cup nonfat peach yogurt
1/2 tsp. cinnamon

Combine orange pieces with marshmallows. Stir cinnamon into peach yogurt, then pour over fruit. Stir to mix. Serve.

153 calories, 0 fat, 2 gm. protein, 36 gm. carbohydrate,
0 cholesterol, 33 mg. sodium, 2.2 gm. dietary fiber,
20 RE vitamin A, 52 mg. vitamin C, 0 vitamin E as
alpha tocopherol

Food exchange
2 1/2 fruit

Preparation time
10 minutes

CITRUS SALAD WITH A KICK

8 servings, 3/4 cup each

4 oranges, peeled and cut into small pieces
2 red grapefruit, peeled and cut into pieces
16-oz. can red kidney beans, drained well
4 ribs celery, sliced thin
1 green onion, sliced thin
1 Tbsp. vegetable oil
1 Tbsp. lemon juice
1/4 cup pineapple juice
1/4 tsp. salt
1/2 tsp. oregano

Combine fruits with kidney beans, celery, and onion in a large salad bowl. In a shaker container, combine remaining ingredients for dressing. Pour dressing over fruits and vegetables, and stir to mix. Refrigerate until serving time.

133 calories, 2 gm. fat, 4 gm. protein, 26 gm. carbohydrate,
0 cholesterol, 303 mg. sodium, 6.8 gm. dietary fiber,
38 RE vitamin A, 68 mg. vitamin C, 0.8 mg. vitamin E as
alpha tocopherol (using sunflower oil)

Food exchange
1 1/2 fruit, 1/2 fat, 1 vegetable

Preparation time
20 minutes

Chilling time
1 hour

COLD SPICED FRUIT

16 servings, 3/4 cup each

1 fresh pineapple
3 fresh peaches
3 fresh pears
1 lb. seedless green grapes
1 cup water
1/2 cup sugar
Thin peelings from 1 orange
1/4 cup orange juice
3 cinnamon sticks
6 whole allspice

Remove crown from pineapple and discard. Peel and cut pineapple into wedges, discarding center core. Cut into 1-inch chunks, and place in a large glass or plastic bowl that has a tight-fitting cover. Core the peaches and pears, and cut into chunks. Add to the pineapple. Add grapes to fruit mixture after removing all stems. In a small saucepan, combine all remaining ingredients. Boil for 3 minutes. Pour over fruit. Mix well, cover, and refrigerate for at least 30 minutes. Remove cinnamon sticks and allspice before serving. This tasty fruit salad keeps in the refrigerator for up to 5 days.

88 calories, 0 fat, 1 gm. protein, 22 gm. carbohydrate, 0 cholesterol, 1 mg. sodium, 1.7 gm. dietary fiber, 13 RE vitamin A, 10 mg. vitamin C, 0 vitamin E as alpha tocopherol

Food exchange
1 1/2 fruit

Preparation time
15 minutes

FIVE-CUP SALAD

10 servings, 1/2 cup each

1 cup crushed pineapple, well drained
1 cup mandarin oranges in juice, well drained
1 cup diced peaches in juice, well drained
1 cup miniature marshmallows
1 cup nonfat sour cream
Garnish: 1/4 cup coconut

Drain fruits well and stir together with marshmallows and sour cream in a salad bowl. Garnish the top of the salad with coconut. Chill for at least 30 minutes or overnight.

81 calories, 0 fat, 1 gm. protein, 18 gm. carbohydrate, 0 cholesterol, 26 mg. sodium, 1 gm. dietary fiber, 25 RE vitamin A, 9 mg. vitamin C, 0 vitamin E as alpha tocopherol

Food exchange
1 1/2 fruit

Preparation time
15 minutes

Chilling time
30 minutes

FROZEN FRUIT SALAD

12 servings, 1/2 cup each

16-oz. bag frozen whole strawberries
20-oz. can crushed pineapple in juice
20-oz. can apricots in juice, quartered
4 fresh bananas, peeled and sliced 1/4- inch thick
12-oz. can sugar-free lemon lime soft drink
Garnish:
1 cup nonfat sour cream
1/2 tsp. vanilla
2 Tbsp. sugar

Combine fruits, their juices, and the soft drink in a large
bowl. Stir to mix, then ladle into muffin cups. Freeze for 6
hours. Meanwhile, combine sour cream with vanilla and
sugar in a small bowl and cover. To remove frozen fruit
cups from the muffin tin, gently dip bottom of muffin tin
in a shallow pan of very hot water. Gently remove each
cup with a spoon. Place each fruit cup in a dish and garnish with sour cream mixture.

140 calories, 1 gm. fat, 2 gm. protein, 31 gm. carbohydrate, 0 cholesterol, 30 mg. sodium, 2.8 gm. dietary fiber, 193 RE vitamin A,
26 mg. vitamin C, 0.3 mg. vitamin E as alpha tocopherol

Food exchange
2 1/2 fruit

Preparation time
15 minutes

Freezing time
6 hours

LATE ALREADY FRUIT SALAD

Need something quick for a potluck or picnic? Stir this together in 5 minutes.

8 servings, 3/4 cup each

13 oz. can chunk, tidbit, or crushed pineapple
16-oz. can apricots in juice
8-oz. can mandarin oranges
3-oz. pkg. instant lemon pudding
1 fresh banana
Garnish: finely grated lime peel

Place a large strainer over a mixing bowl. Drain all fruits well, reserving juice in the bowl. Add pudding to the juices and whisk smooth. Add fruits and sliced banana and chill or serve.

87 calories, 0 fat, 1 gm. protein, 20 gm. carbohydrate, 2 mg. cholesterol, 52 mg. sodium, 2.2 gm. dietary fiber, 114 RE vitamin A, 17 mg. vitamin C, 0.4 mg. vitamin E as alpha tocopherol

Food exchange
1 1/2 fruit

Preparation time
10 minutes

MANDARIN SALAD WITH CRUNCH

8 servings, 3/4 cup each

2 11-oz. cans mandarin oranges
1/2 cup chopped dates
1/4 cup chopped walnuts
3 ribs celery, finely chopped
1/2 cup reduced-fat mayonnaise
Garnish: twisted orange rind

Thouroughly drain the mandarin oranges, reserving 1/3 cup of the juice. Combine drained oranges, dates, walnuts, and celery in a salad bowl. In a small cup or bowl, stir 1/3 cup of the reserved juice into mayonnaise, blending until no lumps remain. Pour dressing over fruit mixture and serve or refrigerate. Garnish salad with a twisted orange rind.

135 calories, 5 gm. fat, 1 gm. protein, 20 gm. carbohydrate, 0 cholesterol, 153 mg. sodium, 1.4 gm. dietary fiber, 14 RE vitamin A, 30 mg. vitamin C, 0 vitamin E as alpha tocopherol

Food exchange
1 fat, 1 1/2 fruit

Preparation time
15 minutes

MARINATED PEARS

8 servings, 3/4 cup each

4 large fresh pears, halved, cored, and sliced
1/4 cup lemon juice
1/4 cup chopped fresh parsley
1/2 tsp. celery seed
1/2 tsp. caraway seed
1/8 tsp. seasoned pepper
1 tsp. vegetable oil

In a large salad bowl, toss pears with remaining ingredients. Marinate for 2 hours in the refrigerator. Serve as a side dish with pork or beef.

58 calories, 0 fat, 0 protein, 13 gm. carbohydrate, 0 cholesterol, 3.2 gm. dietary fiber, 38 RE vitamin A, 14 mg. vitamin C, 0.4 mg. vitamin E as alpha tocopherol

Food exchange
1 fruit

Preparation time
15 minutes

Marinating time
2 hours

MOLDED COTTAGE CHEESE FRUIT SALAD

8 servings, 3/4 cup each

1 3-oz. pkg. sugar-free lemon gelatin
1 3-oz. pkg. sugar-free lime gelatin
1 cup boiling water
1 20-oz. can crushed pineapple, well-drained
1 tsp. horseradish
1/2 cup nonfat sour cream
1/2 cup reduced-fat salad dressing
1 cup nonfat cottage cheese
2 drops green food coloring
Garnish: 1 Tbsp. chopped pecans

In a 3-quart bowl, combine gelatin mixes with boiling water. Stir to dissolve. Add all remaining ingredients and stir well. Transfer to an 8-inch square pan. Garnish with chopped nuts. Chill until firm, about 3 hours, and then cut into 8 pieces.

135 calories, 5 gm. fat, 5 gm. protein, 17 gm. carbohydrate, 2 mg. cholesterol, 235 mg. sodium, 1.4 gm. dietary fiber, 2 9 RE vitamin A, 7 mg. vitamin C, 0 vitamin E as alpha tocopherol

Food exchange
1 fat, 1 fruit, 1/2 lean meat

Preparation time
15 minutes

Chilling time
3 hours

MOLDED CRANBERRY SALAD

8 servings, 1/8 of pan each

1 cup water
1/4 cup sugar
1 lb. cranberries, washed and cleaned
2 3-oz. pkg. sugar-free raspberry gelatin
6 large ice cubes
4 ribs celery, chopped fine
1 large Granny Smith apple, grated with
   peeling on
1 Tbsp. finely grated orange peel

In a medium saucepan, combine water, sugar, and cranberries. Bring to a boil and cook for 5 minutes. Stir in gelatin, then remove pan from heat and continue stirring until gelatin is fully dissolved. Add ice cubes. When ice cubes have melted, stir in celery, grated apple, and orange peel; transfer to 7- by 11-inch casserole dish. Refrigerate for 2 hours or until mixture is set.

45 calories, 0 fat, 0 protein, 12 gm. carbohydrate, 0 cholesterol, 17 mg. sodium, 1.4 gm. dietary fiber, 4 RE vitamin A, 5 mg. vitamin C, 0 vitamin E as alpha tocopherol

Food exchange
1 fruit

Preparation time
15 minutes

Chilling time
3 hours

NUTTY WALDORF SALAD

8 servings, 3/4 cup each

1 lb. green seedless grapes, washed and halved
2 large red apples, cored and cubed
1/2 cup seedless raisins
1/4 cup chopped walnuts
2 ribs celery, diced fine
1/2 cup reduced-fat mayonnaise
1/2 cup nonfat vanilla yogurt
3 or 4 deep green outer romaine lettuce leaves,
    chopped

Combine first five ingredients in a large salad bowl. In a small glass cup, stir together mayonnaise and yogurt. Pour over fruits and stir to mix. Serve this salad on a bed of chopped greens.

163 calories, 6 gm. fat, 2 gm. protein, 27 gm. carbohydrate, 0 cholesterol, 160 mg. sodium, 2.2 gm. dietary fiber, 17 RE vitamin A, 6 mg. vitamin C, 0.3 mg. vitamin E as alpha tocopherol

Food exchange
1 fat, 2 fruit

Preparation time
15 minutes

STRAWBERRY CANTALOUPE SUNDAE

**8 servings, 1/2 cup fruit and yogurt mixture
and 1/8 cantaloupe each**

1 pint fresh strawberries
1 cup grapes
2 bananas, cut into 1/4-inch slices
1 cup vanilla yogurt
1 cantaloupe, cut into eighths

In a mixing bowl, combine fruits with yogurt. Cut cantaloupe in half, remove seeds and then further slice into 8 parts. Place cantaloupe slices on a salad plate. Top with fruit and yogurt mixture.

96 calories, 1 gm. fat, 2 gm. protein, 21 gm. carbohydrate,
3 mg. cholesterol, 19 mg. sodium, 1.6 gm. dietary fiber,
229 RE vitamin A, 53 mg. vitamin C, 0 vitamin E as
alpha tocopherol

Food exchange
1 1/2 fruit

Preparation time
15 minutes

VEGETABLE SALADS

ANY VEGETABLE PASTA SALAD

8 servings, 1 cup each

1 qt. chicken broth
1 1/2 cups your favorite dry pasta
4 cups fresh vegetables of choice (try combination
  of pieces of broccoflower, celery, yellow or red
  pepper, and whole pea pods)
2/3 cup reduced-fat buttermilk ranch dressing
Garnish: dill weed and cherry tomatoes

In a saucepan, bring chicken broth to a boil. Add your
favorite pasta to boiling broth, and cook for 8 minutes.
Immediately drain and rinse pasta with cold water. Prepare
fresh vegetables while pasta is cooking. In a large bowl, combine drained and cooled pasta with vegetables and dressing.
Garnish the top with dill weed and halved cherry tomatoes.

145 calories, 5 gm. fat, 4 gm. protein, 19 gm. carbohydrate, 20 mg.
cholesterol, 878 mg. sodium, (to reduce sodium use reduced-sodium
chicken broth), 1.6 gm. dietary fiber, 14 RE vitamin A,
48 mg. vitamin C, 0 vitamin E as alpha tocopherol

Food exchange
1 fat, 1 bread/starch, 1 vegetable

Preparation time
15 minutes

Cooking time
10 minutes

BACON CAULIFLOWER SALAD

8 servings, 1 cup each

1 head lettuce
1 small head cauliflower
1 red onion
8 strips bacon, diced fine, cooked crisp, and
   drained well
1/4 cup sugar
2/3 cup reduced-fat mayonnaise
1/4 cup grated Parmesan cheese
1/2 tsp. cracked black pepper

Break up lettuce and cauliflower into bite-sized pieces.
Slice and separate onion into thin rings. In a salad bowl,
layer the ingredients in this order: lettuce, onion rings,
bacon, and cauliflower. Combine remaining ingredients,
and spread over the top. Cover tightly and chill overnight.
Mix well before serving.

185 calories, 9 gm. fat, 7 gm. protein, 19 gm. carbohydrate,
7 mg. cholesterol, 414 mg. sodium, 0 dietary fiber, 51 RE vitamin A,
62 mg. vitamin C, 0 vitamin E as alpha tocopherol

Food exchange
2 fat, 4 vegetable

Preparation time
15 minutes

Chilling time
6 to 8 hours

FIVE-BEAN SALAD WITH PEPPER AND PIMIENTO

16 servings, 1 cup each

16-oz. can kitchen cut green beans, drained well
17-oz. can lima beans, drained well
16-oz. can kidney beans, drained well
16-oz. can wax beans, drained well
15-oz. can garbanzo beans, drained well
1 large green pepper, chopped
2-oz. jar sliced pimiento, drained
2 Tbsp. minced dried onion
2 cups vinegar
2 cups sugar
1 tsp. salt
4 large ice cubes

Drain all beans well and place in a large bowl. Add pepper and pimiento. In a large saucepan, combine dried onion, vinegar, sugar, and salt and bring to a boil. Reduce heat and simmer for 3 minutes. Remove from heat, add 4 large ice cubes, stir to melt, and then pour over beans. Stir to mix. Refrigerate for at least 2 hours. This salad keeps well for up to 7 days.

◆

228 calories, 1 gm. fat, 8 gm. protein, 49 gm. carbohydrate, 0 cholesterol, 435 mg. sodium, 6.5 gm. dietary fiber, 26 RE vitamin A, 18 mg. vitamin C, 0 vitamin E as alpha tocopherol

Food exchange
3 vegetable, 2 bread/starch

Preparation time
15 minutes

Chilling time
2 hours

BROCCOLI SLAW

8 servings, 3/4 cup each

1 yellow pepper, diced
1-lb. bag broccoli coleslaw mix
1 Tbsp. vegetable oil
3 Tbsp. red wine vinegar
1 tsp. prepared mustard
1/2 tsp. salt
1/2 tsp. caraway seeds
1/4 tsp. black pepper

In a large salad bowl, combine diced yellow pepper and broccoli. In a shaker container, mix remaining ingredients until well blended. Pour dressing over vegetables, toss gently, and serve immediately.

54 calories, 2 gm. fat, 3 gm. protein, 8 gm. carbohydrate, 0 cholesterol, 172 mg. sodium, 3.6 gm. dietary fiber, 181 RE vitamin A, 157 mg. vitamin C, 0.8 mg. vitamin E as alpha tocopherol (using sunflower oil)

Food exchange
1 vegetable, 1/2 fat

Preparation time
15 minutes

CARROT PINEAPPLE SALAD

8 servings, 3/4 cup each

1 lb. carrots, scrubbed well and shredded
8-oz. can crushed pineapple, well drained
1/4 cup golden raisins
1 cup nonfat pineapple yogurt
Garnish: carrot tops

In a salad bowl, combine shredded carrots with pineapple and raisins. Fold in yogurt. Garnish the bowl with carrot tops and serve.

74 calories, 0 fat, 2 gm. protein, 16 gm. carbohydrate, 1 mg. cholesterol, 40 mg. sodium, 1.8 gm. dietary fiber, 1593 RE vitamin A, 7 mg. vitamin C, 0 vitamin E as alpha tocopherol

Food exchange
1 vegetable, 1 fruit

Preparation time
20 minutes

CHILLED BRUSSELS SPROUTS SALAD

8 servings, 3/4 cup each

16 oz. frozen brussels sprouts
1 lb. zucchini, sliced thin
1 red onion, peeled and sliced thin
2/3 cup reduced-fat Italian dressing
1/2 tsp. finely grated fresh lemon peel

In a microwave-safe casserole dish, combine frozen brussels sprouts with sliced zucchini. Cover and microcook on high power for 6 minutes. Use a slotted spoon to transfer vegetables to a salad bowl. Sprinkle with onion slices, and then Italian dressing. Cover and chill for 2 hours. Sprinkle with finely grated fresh lemon peel just before serving.

62 calories, 2 gm. fat, 3 gm. protein, 9 gm. carbohydrate, 1 mg. cholesterol, 164 mg. sodium, 2.8 gm. dietary fiber, 52 RE vitamin A, 32 mg. vitamin C, 0 vitamin E as alpha tocopherol

Food exchange
2 vegetable, 1 fat

Preparation time
15 minutes

MicroCooking time
6 minutes

Chilling time
2 hours

CHILLED SWEET AND SOUR MIXED VEGETABLE SALAD

8 servings, 3/4 cup each

8 ribs celery, diced fine
1 small red onion, chopped fine
16-oz. pkg. frozen mixed vegetables, thawed
1/2 cup sugar
1/3 cup vinegar
2 Tbsp. prepared mustard
2 tsp. flour

Combine celery, red onion, and mixed vegetables in a large salad bowl. In a small saucepan, combine remaining ingredients for dressing, using a whisk to blend. Over medium heat, bring mixture to a boil for 1 minute, then remove pan from heat. Cool dressing. To speed cooling, transfer dressing to a chilled metal bowl and stir to promote dissipation of heat. Pour dressing over vegetables, stirring well. Cover and refrigerate until serving.

126 calories, 0 fat, 3 gm. protein, 0 cholesterol, 132 mg. sodium, 5.8 gm. dietary fiber, 489 RE vitamin A, 7 mg. vitamin C, 0 vitamin E as alpha tocopherol

Food exchange
2 vegetable, 1 1/2 fruit

Preparation time
15 minutes

CLASSIC BEAN SALAD

This salad is a never-fail quick side dish for soups and sandwiches.

8 servings, 3/4 cup each

16-oz. can green beans, well drained
16-oz. can red kidney beans, well drained
16-oz. can wax beans, well-drained
1 large white onion, chopped fine
1 Tbsp. vegetable oil
3/4 cup vinegar
1/4 cup sugar
1 tsp. salt
1/2 tsp. black pepper

In a salad bowl, mix drained beans with onion. Mix all remaining ingredients in a shaker container. Pour dressing over beans and stir carefully. Serve immediately or refrigerate for up to 3 days.

183 calories, 1 gm. fat, 10 gm. protein, 33 gm. carbohydrate, 0 cholesterol, 319 mg. sodium, 4.5 gm. dietary fiber, 10 RE vitamin A, 4 mg. vitamin C, 0.8 mg. vitamin E as alpha tocopherol (using sunflower oil)

Food exchange
1 vegetable, 2 bread/starch

Preparation time
15 minutes

CORN RELISH SALAD WITH DILL

8 servings, 3/4 cup each

2 16-oz. cans whole-kernel corn, well drained
4 ribs celery, sliced diagonally
1 small red pepper, chopped
1/4 cup chopped pimiento
1/2 tsp. dill weed
1/8 cup vegetable oil
1/4 cup vinegar
1 tsp. sugar
1/2 tsp. salt
1/2 tsp. paprika
1/2 tsp. dry mustard
3 drops hot sauce

Drain corn well and mix in a salad bowl with celery, pepper, and pimiento. In a shaker container, combine remaining ingredients. Pour over corn mixture, cover, and refrigerate for at least 30 minutes to allow flavors to blend.

132 calories, 4 gm. fat, 3 gm. protein, 23 gm. carbohydrate, 0 cholesterol, 151 mg. sodium, 3.6 gm. dietary fiber, 38 RE vitamin A, 32 mg. vitamin C, 1.5 mg. vitamin E as alpha tocopherol (using sunflower oil)

Food exchange
1 bread/starch, 1 vegetable, 1/2 fat

Preparation time
15 minutes

Chilling time
30 minutes

CREAMY COLESLAW

8 servings, 3/4 cup each

1-lb. bag of shredded cabbage
1 large green pepper, diced
2/3 cup reduced-fat mayonnaise
2 Tbsp. cider vinegar
1/2 tsp. salt
1/2 tsp. lemon juice
1/4 tsp. black pepper
2 tsp. sugar

In a salad bowl, combine shredded cabbage and diced pepper. Combine remaining ingredients in a small mixing bowl, blending smooth. Pour dressing over cabbage. Allow to chill for 1 hour if time permits.

89 calories, 6 gm. fat, 1 gm. protein, 7 gm. carbohydrate, 0 cholesterol, 282 mg. sodium, 1 gm. dietary fiber, 26 RE vitamin A, 43 mg. vitamin C, 0.9 mg. vitamin E as alpha tocopherol

Food exchange
2 vegetable, 1 fat

Preparation time
15 minutes

Optional chilling time
1 hour

CUCUMBER CARROT SALAD

8 servings, 1 cup each

5 large carrots, sliced into coins
2 Tbsp. water
6 large ice cubes
1 large green pepper, diced
1 large onion, chopped fine
1 cucumber, sliced thin
4 ribs celery, diced fine
6-oz. can tomato paste
1 Tbsp. prepared mustard
1/2 cup brown sugar
2/3 cup vinegar

In a microwave-safe casserole dish, combine sliced carrots and 2 tablespoons of water. Cover and microwave on high power for 6 minutes. Transfer the steamed carrots to a salad bowl, and put ice cubes over the hot carrots to speed cooling. Drain water from carrots. Add green pepper, onion, cucumber, and celery to the salad bowl and stir to mix. In a glass cup, combine tomato paste, mustard, brown sugar, and vinegar. Heat in the microwave for up to 2 minutes, just until the brown sugar is fully dissolved. Pour over vegetables, mix, and refrigerate for at least 2 hours before serving. This salad can be refrigerated for up to 3 days.

119 calories, 0 fat, 2 gm. protein, 29 gm. carbohydrate, 0 cholesterol, 78 mg. sodium, 2.4 gm. dietary fiber, 1346 RE vitamin A, 43 mg. vitamin C, 0 vitamin E as alpha tocopherol

Food exchange
1 vegetable, 1 fruit

Preparation time
10 minutes

Chilling time
2 hours

DONNA'S HERBED TOMATOES

This recipe is a favorite during tomato season and is shared with permission of my friend Donna Borcherding.

8 servings, 1/2 tomato each

4 large ripe, but firm, tomatoes
2/3 cup reduced-fat Italian dressing
Garnish:
2 Tbsp. fresh parsley, minced, and
2 Tbsp. Parmesan cheese

Use a serrated knife to carefully cut tomatoes into 1/2-inch slices. Place in a shallow pan and pour dressing over them. Cover the pan and refrigerate at least 2 hours or overnight. Chill salad plates, then place 3 slices of tomato on each plate. Garnish with minced parsley and Parmesan cheese and serve. This is an excellent side dish to a soup and bread luncheon.

51 calories, 3 gm. fat, 2 gm. protein, 4 gm. carbohydrate, 5 mg. cholesterol, 213 mg. sodium, 0.5 gm. dietary fiber, 63 RE vitamin A, 16 mg. vitamin C, 1.5 mg. vitamin E as alpha tocopherol

Food exchange
1/2 fat, 1 vegetable

Preparation time
15 minutes

Chilling time
2 hours or overnight

ELEGANT ASPARAGUS VINAIGRETTE

8 servings, 1 cup each

2 lb. fresh asparagus
2 Tbsp. water
8 ice cubes
1/4 cup Dijon-style mustard
2 Tbsp. wine vinegar
1/4 tsp. salt
1/4 tsp. white pepper
1 tsp. dried tarragon

Wash asparagus well, then snap off white ends of asparagus spears. Cut away any dried or tough spikes. Cut the spears into 4-inch long pieces. Place in a microwave-safe container, sprinkle with water, and cover. Microcook for 4 minutes. Remove from the oven, uncover, and toss with ice cubes to stop the cooking process. When ice cubes are melted, drain water from the vegetables and save it for soup or a cold vegetable juice cocktail. Meanwhile, in a shaker container, combine all remaining ingredients. Pour over cooled asparagus and refrigerate until well chilled—at least 30 minutes.

32 calories, 0 fat, 3 gm. protein, 4 gm. carbohydrate, 0 cholesterol, 160 mg. sodium, 3.6 gm. dietary fiber, 101 RE vitamin A, 37 mg. vitamin C, 5.5 mg. vitamin E as alpha tocopherol

Food exchange
1 vegetable

Preparation time
10 minutes

GREEN AND WHITE POTATO SALAD

8 servings, 3/4 cup each

4 large potatoes
1/4 cup water
1/2 cup white wine
1 14-oz. can no-added-salt French-style green
    beans, well-drained
1/2 cup reduced-fat French dressing
2 Tbsp. chopped fresh parsley
1/4 tsp. white pepper

Peel potatoes if desired. Cut into 1/2-inch cubes and place in a microwave-safe casserole dish. Sprinkle with 1/4 cup water, cover, and microcook on high power for 8 minutes. Stir twice during cooking. When potatoes are tender, drain, and douse with chilled white wine. Stir to speed cooling. As soon as the potatoes are cool enough to handle, drain well and discard wine. Add well-drained beans, French dressing, parsley, and pepper; stir carefully. Chill for at least 30 minutes or until serving time.

140 calories, 1 gm. fat, 3 gm. protein, 28 gm. carbohydrate, 0 cholesterol, 252 mg. sodium, 3.4 gm. dietary fiber, 36 RE vitamin A, 21 mg. vitamin C, 1 mg. vitamin E as alpha tocopherol
(from salad dressing)

Food exchange
1 1/2 bread/starch, 2 vegetable

Preparation time
20 minutes

HEARTS OF PALM GREEN SALAD

This pale, tender vegetable has a delicate flavor and texture resembling an artichoke heart. It is harvested from the palm tree.

8 servings, 1 cup each

14-oz. can hearts of palm, drained
6 cups chopped romaine lettuce
1 medium tomato, cut into wedges
6 large radishes, sliced thin
2 Tbsp. vinegar
1/2 tsp. tarragon
1 Tbsp. vegetable oil
2 tsp. Dijon-style mustard
1/4 tsp. garlic powder

Combine first four ingredients in a large salad bowl. In a shaker container, combine remaining ingredients and shake until well mixed. Pour dressing over vegetables just before serving.

57 calories, 2 gm. fat, 3 gm. protein, 7 gm. carbohydrate, 0 cholesterol, 38 mg. sodium, 1.2 gm. dietary fiber, 459 RE vitamin A, 60 mg. vitamin C, 0 vitamin E as alpha tocopherol

Food exchange
1 vegetable, 1/2 fat

Preparation time
15 minutes

JICAMA SLAW

This is tasty with grilled white fish.

8 servings, 3/4 cup each

2 large jicamas, peeled and grated
4 large carrots, scrubbed well and grated
2 Granny Smith apples, grated
1/2 tsp. garlic powder
1/4 cup vinegar
1 Tbsp. vegetable oil
2 tsp. prepared mustard
1/4 cup apple juice
1/4 tsp. salt
1/4 tsp. black pepper

Combine jicama, carrots, and apples in a salad bowl. In a shaker container, mix remaining ingredients for dressing. Pour dressing over slaw just before serving.

95 calories, 1 gm. fat, 3 gm. protein, 18 gm. carbohydrate,
0 cholesterol, 74 mg. sodium, 2.8 gm. dietary fiber,
1518 RE vitamin A, 9 mg. vitamin C,
0 vitamin E as alpha tocopheral

Food exchange
1 vegetable, 1 fruit

Preparation time
20 minutes

KOHLRABI SLAW

8 servings, 3/4 cup each

6 medium kohlrabies
2 red apples, cored and chopped; reserve 3 slices
for garnish
1 green onion, sliced thin; reserve tops
1/2 cup nonfat sour cream
1/4 cup reduced-fat western-style dressing
1/2 tsp. celery seed

Peel kohlrabies and shred into a medium salad bowl. Add
chopped apples and green onion. In a small bowl, combine sour cream, western-style dressing, and celery seed.
Add dressing to vegetables and chill for up to one hour
or serve immediately. Garnish salad with green onion
tops alternated with red apple slices, forming a fan in the
middle of the salad.

84 calories, 1 gm. fat, 3 gm. protein, 17 gm. carbohydrate, 1 mg.
cholesterol, 161 mg. sodium, 2.2 gm. dietary fiber, 25 RE vitamin A,
73 mg. vitamin C, 0 vitamin E as alpha tocopherol

Food exchange
1 fruit, 1 vegetable

Preparation time
20 minutes

Optional chilling time
up to 1 hour

KRAUT SALAD

8 servings, 1 cup each

1 16-oz. can sauerkraut, reserving 1/4 cup liquid
    after draining well
1 rib celery, finely chopped
1 green onion, diced
3 large carrots, shredded
2/3 cup sugar or equivalent sugar substitute
1/4 cup vinegar

Drain sauerkraut and snip into bite sized pieces. Combine kraut with celery, onion, and carrot in a medium salad bowl. Combine reserved sauerkraut juice, sugar, and vinegar in a small saucepan. Bring to a boil, stirring constantly. Remove from heat and pour over vegetables. Toss to coat. Chill for at least 2 hours or up to 3 days.

90 calories (60 with sugar substitute), 0 fat, 0 protein, 22 gm. carbohydrate (15 gm. with sugar substitute), 0 cholesterol, 389 mg. sodium, 2.4 gm. dietary fiber, 763 RE vitamin A, 12 mg. vitamin C, 0 vitamin E as alpha tocopherol

Food exchange
1 vegetable, 1 fruit
(1 vegetable, 1/2 fruit with sugar substitute)

Preparation time
15 minutes

MAKE YOUR OWN BUTTERMILK RANCH DRESSING

16 servings, 1 tablespoon each

1/2 cup reduced-fat mayonnaise
1/2 cup buttermilk
2 tsp. dried parsley flakes
1 1/2 tsp. dried onion
1/2 tsp. salt
1/4 tsp. celery salt
1/4 tsp. garlic powder

Mix all ingredients in a shaker container and store in the refrigerator for use with green salads. This keeps for a month.

35 calories, 3 gm. fat, 0 protein, 2 gm. carbohydrate, 0 cholesterol, 198 mg. sodium, 0 dietary fiber, 1 RE vitamin A, 0 vitamin E as alpha tocopherol

Food exchange
1 fat

Preparation time
15 minutes

Chilling time
3 hour

MARINATED MUSHROOM SIDE SALAD

8 servings, 1/2 cup each

1 Tbsp. vegetable oil
2/3 cup white vinegar
1/4 cup water
1/4 tsp. garlic powder
1 bay leaf
10 peppercorns
1 tsp. dill seed
1/4 tsp. salt
1 lb. fresh mushrooms

Mix oil, vinegar, and water in a medium saucepan. Add garlic, bay leaf, peppercorns, dill seed, and salt. Cover and simmer for 10 minutes. Meanwhile, clean mushrooms with a paper towel. Slice mushrooms lengthwise, including stem, into a ceramic salad bowl. Pour hot marinade over mushrooms; stir to mix. Cover and refrigerate for at least 2 hours. Serve as a side dish with red meats or as a topping on fresh greens.

32 calories, 1 gm. fat, 2 gm. protein, 3 gm. carbohydrate,
0 cholesterol, 68 mg. sodium, 0.4 gm. dietary fiber, 0 RE vitamin A,
1 mg. vitamin C, 0 vitamin E as alpha tocopherol

Food exchange
1 vegetable

Preparation time
15 minutes

Marinating time
2 hours

MEXICAN COLESLAW

8 servings, 1 cup each

1-lb. bag shredded cabbage
3 ribs celery, finely cut
1 large banana pepper, diced
1/4 cup sugar
1 tsp. salt
2 Tbsp. vegetable oil
1/4 cup water
1/3 cup vinegar
Garnish: 1/4 cup chopped pimiento

Combine cabbage, celery, and diced pepper in a salad bowl.
In a shaker container, combine sugar, salt, oil, water, and
vinegar until sugar is fully dissolved. Pour dressing over
vegetables and mix well. Garnish the top of the salad with
chopped pimiento. Chill until serving time.

77 calories, 3 gm. fat, 1 gm. protein, 11 gm. carbohydrate, 0 cholesterol, 290 mg. sodium, 2.7 gm. dietary fiber, 32 RE vitamin A,
46 mg. vitamin C, 0 vitamin E as alpha tocopherol

Food exchange
1/2 fat, 2 vegetable

Preparation time
15 minutes

OLD-FASHIONED PEA SALAD

8 servings, 3/4 cup each

16-oz. bag frozen green peas, thawed and drained
  well
2 oz. reduced-fat cheddar cheese, cubed
2 hard-boiled egg whites, chopped
2 ribs celery, chopped fine
1 very small white onion, chopped
1/3 cup reduced-fat mayonnaise
1/4 tsp. salt
1/4 tsp. Tabasco® sauce
1/8 tsp. black pepper
Garnish: paprika

In a medium salad bowl, combine peas, cheese cubes, egg whites, celery, and onion. In a small mixing bowl, combine remaining ingredients for dressing. Fold dressing into the pea mixture. Refrigerate up to overnight or serve immediately. Garnish with paprika.

112 calories, 5 gm. fat, 6 gm. protein, 10 gm. carbohydrate, 5 mg. cholesterol, 264 mg. sodium, 1.4 gm. dietary fiber, 63 RE vitamin A, 6 mg. vitamin C, 0 vitamin E as alpha tocopherol

Food exchange
1 vegetable, 1/2 bread/starch, 1 fat

Preparation time
15 minutes

ORIENTAL PEA POD SALAD

8 servings, 1 cup each

16-oz. bag frozen stir-fry vegetables
3 cups finely sliced bok choy
1 cup bean sprouts
1 Tbsp. vegetable oil
1/3 cup vinegar
2 Tbsp. sugar
1 Tbsp. reduced-sodium soy sauce
1/8 tsp. black pepper

Thaw frozen vegetables in a colander until they are soft and well drained. Place in a salad bowl, and add chopped bok choy and bean sprouts. Combine remaining ingredients in a shaker container and pour over the salad; toss and serve.

91 calories, 2 gm. fat, 3 gm. protein, 17 gm. carbohydrate, 0 cholesterol, 163 mg. sodium, 1.2 gm. dietary fiber, 272 RE vitamin A, 54 mg. vitamin C, 0 vitamin E as alpha tocopherol

Food exchange
1/2 fat, 2 vegetable, 1/2 fruit

Preparation time
15 minutes

PERFECTION SALAD

8 servings, 3/4 cup each

2 3-oz. pkg. sugar-free lemon-flavored gelatin
3 cups water, divide
1/3 cup vinegar
2 Tbsp. lemon juice
2 cups shredded cabbage
1/2 cup shredded carrots
1/2 cup chopped celery
1/2 cup chopped green pepper
Garnish: reduced fat mayonnaise

Combine lemon gelatin and 2 cups boiling water in a mixing bowl. Stir to completely dissolve gelatin. Stir in remaining 1 cup cold water, vinegar, and lemon juice. Chill mixture for 30 minutes. Fold in vegetables and turn mixture into a 6-cup mold or an 8-inch square dish. Chill until set, at least 1 1/2 hours. Place molded salad on a plate lined with lettuce. Garnish with reduced-fat mayonnaise at serving time.

32 calories, 0 fat, 1 gm. protein, 7 gm. carbohydrate, 0 cholesterol, 32 mg. sodium, 0.8 gm. dietary fiber, 810 RE vitamin A, 28 mg. vitamin C, 0 vitamin E as alpha tocopherol

Food exchange
1 vegetable

Preparation time
10 minutes

Chilling time
2 hours

PICKLED BEET SALAD

16 servings, 3/4 cup each

2 lb. fresh beets, cooked, peeled, and diced
3 large apples, peeled, cored, and diced
1 large onion, diced
1 cinnamon stick, broken
1/3 cup sugar or equivalent in sugar substitute
1 cup vinegar
1 tsp. salt

Combine diced beets, apples, and onions in a salad bowl. In a small saucepan, combine all remaining ingredients. Cook over medium heat for 5 minutes, until sugar is fully dissolved. Remove cinnamon stick, then pour the mixture over the apples and beets. To speed cooling, add 4 ice cubes. Refrigerate for at least 30 minutes before serving. This salad keeps for up to a week.

120 calories with sugar (90 with sugar substitute), 0 fat, 2 gm. protein, 32 gm. carbohydrate with sugar (24 gm. with sugar substitute), 0 cholesterol, 122 mg. sodium, 3.3 gm. dietary fiber, 9 RE vitamin A, 13 mg. vitamin C, 0.9 mg. vitamin E as alpha tocopherol

Food exchange
2 fruit
(1 1/2 fruit with sugar substitute)

Preparation time
15 minutes

Cooking time
5 minutes

Chilling time:
30 minutes

POTATO SALAD WITH SOUR CREAM DRESSING

16 servings, 3/4 cup each

6 large potatoes, peeled, boiled, and chopped
3 eggs, hard boiled and sliced
4 ribs celery, thinly sliced
1 yellow onion, diced
1 cup nonfat sour cream
1/2 cup reduced-fat mayonnaise
3 Tbsp. vinegar
1 tsp. salt
1/4 tsp. pepper
1 Tbsp. dill pickle relish

In a salad bowl, combine potatoes and eggs with celery and onion. Combine sour cream with remaining ingredients in a small mixing bowl. Pour dressing over potatoes and fold to blend. Refrigerate until ready to serve.

100 calories, 3 gm. fat, 3 gm. protein, 14 gm. carbohydrate, 42 mg. cholesterol, 252 mg. sodium, 1.4 gm. dietary fiber, 33 RE vitamin A, 6 mg. vitamin C, 0 vitamin E as alpha tocopherol

Food exchange
1/2 fat, 1 bread/starch

Preparation time
15 minutes

Potato/egg Cooking time
25 minutes

RED CABBAGE SLAW

12 servings, 1 cup each

1 large head red cabbage, shredded
4 green onions, diced
1/4 cup almonds
1/4 cup raisins
4 large carrots, shredded
2/3 cup reduced-fat mayonnaise
1/2 cup nonfat sour cream
2 Tbsp. vinegar
1 tsp. dill seed
1 tsp. caraway seed
1/2 tsp. salt
1/2 tsp. white pepper

In a large salad bowl, combine cabbage, onions, almonds, raisins, and carrots. In a small mixing bowl, whisk remaining ingredients until no lumps remain. Pour dressing over salad up to 1 hour before serving, mix well and refrigerate until serving.

115 calories, 7 gm. fat, 3 gm. protein, 12 gm. carbohydrate, 4 mg. cholesterol, 228 mg. sodium, 2.4 gm. dietary fiber, 685 RE vitamin A, 30 mg. vitamin C, 2.2 mg. vitamin E as alpha tocopherol (from almonds)

Food exchange
1 fat, 1/2 fruit, 2 vegetable

Preparation time
20 minutes

Chilling time
1 hour

SANDY'S SPINACH AND APPLE SALAD

8 servings, 2 cups each

2 bunches fresh spinach
1 large Red Delicious apple, cored and sliced thin
1/4 cup chopped red onion
1 cup chopped celery
1/4 cup whole walnuts or pecans
1/2 cup sugar
1/3 cup vinegar
2 Tbsp. finely-grated white onion
1 tsp. dry mustard
1/8 cup vegetable oil (try sunflower or safflower)
1 1/2 Tbsp. poppy seed

Wash spinach, drain well, and tear into bite-sized pieces. Combine with apple, onion, celery, and nuts in a large salad bowl. In a shaker container, combine remaining ingredients for the dressing, mixing well. Pour dressing over the salad just before serving. The dressing keeps for several weeks in the refrigerator.

171 calories, 8 gm. fat, 4 gm. protein, 22 gm. carbohydrate, 0 cholesterol, 114 mg. sodium, 2.8 gm. dietary fiber, 765 RE vitamin A, 35 mg. vitamin C, 1.7 mg. vitamin E as alpha tocopherol

Food exchange
1 1/2 fat, 1 fruit, 2 vegetable

Preparation time
15 minutes

SEVEN-LAYER SALAD

8 servings, 1 cup each

1 bag spinach, washed and torn into small pieces
2 ribs celery, sliced fine
1 large red pepper, chopped fine
2 scallions, chopped fine
10 oz. frozen peas, thawed
1 cup reduced-fat mayonnaise
1 Tbsp. sugar
2 oz. reduced-fat cheddar cheese, shredded
2 oz. lean ham, diced into small cubes

Layer first five ingredients in order listed in an 11- by 7-inch pan. In a glass measuring cup, mix the mayonnaise with the sugar. Spread over the peas. Sprinkle cheese and ham on top. Cover and refrigerate for 2 hours or overnight. Use a spatula or large spoon to serve the salad.

195 calories, 11 gm. fat, 9 gm. protein, 15 gm. carbohydrate, 17 mg. cholesterol, 449 mg. sodium, 1.8 gm. dietary fiber, 808 RE vitamin A, 90 mg. vitamin C, 0.5 mg. vitamin E as alpha tocopherol

Food exchange
2 fat, 1/2 lean meat, 2 vegetable, 1/2 bread/starch

Preparation time
20 minutes

Chilling time
2 to 8 hours

SHOE PEG SALAD

8 servings, 3/4 oz. each

16-oz. can white peg corn, drained well
4 scallions, chopped fine (including tops)
1 green pepper, finely chopped
1 3-oz. jar diced pimientos
2 stalks celery, finely chopped
6 oz. frozen peas, thawed
1/3 cup vinegar
1/4 cup oil
1/4 cup sugar

Mix first six ingredients in a large salad bowl. In a shaker container, mix vinegar, oil, and sugar until clear. Pour over salad and mix well. Chill until ready to serve. This salad keeps for up to 5 days in the refrigerator.

163 calories, 7 gm. fat, 3 gm. protein, 24 gm. carbohydrate, 0 cholesterol, 29 mg. sodium, 4.8 gm. dietary fiber, 65 RE vitamin A, 36 mg. vitamin C, 0 vitamin E as alpha tocopherol

Food exchange
1 fat, 1 bread/starch, 1 vegetable

Preparation time
20 minutes

SPINACH SALAD WITH BLUE CHEESE AND BACON

16 servings, 1 cup each

1 cup reduced-fat chunky blue cheese dressing
1 cup nonfat sour cream
2 green onions, finely chopped
4 slices bacon, cooked crisp, drained, and crumbled
1 bag fresh spinach, washed and torn into small
    pieces (about 10 oz.)
1 cup cauliflowerets
1 cup shredded carrots
8 cherry tomatoes, halved
1 medium cucumber, sliced thin
1/2 small head red cabbage, finely shredded

In a medium bowl, blend dressing, sour cream, green
onions, and bacon. In a 2-quart salad bowl, layer half of
the spinach, cauliflower, carrots, tomatoes, remaining
spinach, cucumber, and cabbage. Spoon dressing over the
salad, cover, and chill for several hours or overnight.

88 calories, 2 gm. fat, 4 gm. protein, 12 gm. carbohydrate,
5 mg. cholesterol, 318 mg. sodium, 1.1 gm. dietary fiber,
1804 RE vitamin A, 40 mg. vitamin C,
1.2 mg. vitamin E as alpha tocopherol

Food exchange
1 fat, 2 vegetable

Preparation time
20 minutes

Chilling time
2 hours

SPINACH SALAD WITH SOY SAUCE DRESSING

8 servings, 1 cup each

1 lb. fresh spinach, washed and torn into small pieces
1 lb. fresh mushrooms, thinly sliced
3 large carrots, scrubbed and grated
2 Tbsp. reduced sodium soy sauce
2 Tbsp. rice vinegar
1 Tbsp. vegetable oil (try sunflower)
2 Tbsp. water
1/4 tsp. ginger
Garnish: crunchy chow mein noodles

Combine spinach with mushrooms and grated carrots in a large salad bowl. In a shaker container, mix together soy sauce, rice vinegar, oil, water, and ginger. Toss dressing with vegetables just before serving. Garnish the top of the salad with chow mein noodles.

56 calories, 2 gm. fat, 3 gm. protein, 7 gm. carbohydrate, 0 cholesterol, 312 mg. sodium, 1.8 gm. dietary fiber, 1139 RE vitamin A, 20 mg. vitamin C, 0.8 mg. vitamin E as alpha tocopherol

Food exchange
1 vegetable, 1/2 fat

Preparation time
10 minutes

STIR-FRY VEGGIE AND WILD RICE SALAD

8 servings, 1 cup each

3 cups water
1 cup dry brown or wild rice (or a mixture
of the two)
16-oz. pkg. frozen stir-fry vegetables
2 ribs celery, diced
2/3 cup reduced-fat honey-Dijon salad dressing
Garnish: sunflower seeds

Bring water to a boil in a medium saucepan. Add rice,
cover, and cook for 25 minutes or until tender. Drain well,
and fluff. Place frozen vegetables in a large salad bowl. Add
cooked rice and stir to mix. The vegetables will speed
cooling of the rice. Add celery to the mixture. Add dressing to the salad just before serving. Garnish with a few
sunflower seeds.

220 calories, 9 gm. fat, 4 gm. protein, 31 gm. carbohydrate, 0 cholesterol, 222 mg. sodium, 2.2 gm. dietary fiber, 243 RE vitamin A,
2 mg. vitamin C, 0 vitamin E as alpha tocopherol

Food exchange
2 bread/starch, 2 fat

Preparation time
10 minutes

Cooking time
25 minutes

SWEET AND SOUR CABBAGE SALAD

8 servings, 1 cup each

1 bag (6 cups) shredded cabbage and carrots
1 red or green bell pepper, chopped
2 green onions, thinly sliced, including tops
1/2 tsp. celery seed
1/2 tsp. mustard seed
1/2 cup water
1/4 cup sugar
1/2 cup vinegar

Combine vegetables and seeds in a large salad bowl. In a small saucepan over high heat, combine water, sugar, and vinegar. Bring to a boil and cook for 2 minutes. Let cool to room temperature. Stir dressing into vegetables; cover and refrigerate for 24 hours. Serve with a slotted spoon. This salad will be tasty for a week when kept refrigerated.

80 calories, 0 fat, 2 gm. protein, 19 gm. carbohydrate, 0 cholesterol, 34 mg. sodium, 2.6 gm. dietary fiber, 1551 RE vitamin A, 5 mg. vitamin C, 0.9 mg. vitamin E as alpha tocopherol

Food exchange
2 vegetable, 1/2 fruit

Preparation time
15 minutes

Marinating time
24 hours

WESTERN SWEET POTATO SALAD

8 servings, 3/4 cup each

6 large sweet potatoes
1/4 cup water
1 medium white onion, cut into thin rings
1 green pepper, cut into thin strips
2/3 cup reduced-fat western-style dressing
1/2 tsp. celery seed

Wash sweet potatoes well. Peel and cut into 1/4-inch thick slices. Place in a microwave-safe casserole dish and sprinkle with 1/4 cup water. Cover and microcook on high power for 8 to 10 minutes, until fork-tender, stopping to stir the potatoes twice during cooking. Transfer the potatoes to a salad bowl. Sprinkle with white onion, green pepper, dressing, and celery seed. Cover and chill for at least 2 hours. Use a large spoon to carefully stir salad before serving. Makes side dish with turkey.

206 calories, 0 fat, 3 gm. protein, 47 gm. carbohydrate, 0 cholesterol, 22 mg. sodium, 6.6 gm. dietary fiber, 1866 RE vitamin A, 55 mg. vitamin C, 4.4 mg. vitamin E as alpha tocopherol

Food exchange
2 1/2 bread/starch

Preparation time
15 minutes

MicroCooking time
10 minutes

Chilling time
2 hours

ZUCCHINI BLEU CHEESE SALAD

8 servings, 3/4 cup each

3 large zucchini, cut in thin slices
1 red pepper, diced
2 carrots, shredded
2/3 cup reduced-fat bleu cheese dressing
Optional garnish: 1/4 cup toasted almonds

In a salad bowl, combine sliced zucchini, diced pepper, and shredded carrots. Fold in dressing, garnish the top of the salad with almonds. Makes a nice side dish with grilled hamburgers.

76 calories, 2 gm. fat, 2 gm. protein, 11 gm. carbohydrate, 5 mg. cholesterol, 314 mg. sodium, 1.8 gm. dietary fiber, 70 RE vitamin A, 69 mg. vitamin C, 3.3 mg. vitamin E as alpha tocopherol (with almonds)

Food exchange
2 vegetable, 1/2 fat

Preparation time
10 minutes

HOT VEGETABLES

CANDIED CARROTS

4 servings, 3/4 cup each

1 lb. fresh carrots
1 Tbsp. water
1/2 cup all-fruit orange marmalade (such as
   Simply Fruit®)
1/2 tsp. cornstarch

Wash carrots very well, using a brush to scrub clean. Peel,
if desired. Cut carrots into coins. Place in a 2-quart casserole dish with 1 tablespoon water. Cover and microcook
on high power for 10 minutes. Combine cornstarch with
marmalade in a small cup, stirring until smooth. Stir marmalade mixture into the carrots, and microcook 3 more
minutes, uncovered.

76 calories, 0 fat, 1 gm. protein, 18 gm. carbohydrate, 0 cholesterol,
60 mg. sodium, 1.2 gm. dietary fiber, 2531 RE vitamin A,
6 mg. vitamin C, 0 vitamin E as alpha tocopherol

Food exchange
1/2 fruit, 2 vegetable

Preparation time
10 minutes

Microcooking time
13 minutes

CAULIFLOWER WITH CHEESE SAUCE

8 servings, 1 cup each

1 medium head cauliflower, cleaned and stem
  removed
2 Tbsp. water
2/3 cup soft spreadable cheese
  (such as Cheeze Whiz®)
1/4 cup skim milk
1 /2 tsp. prepared mustard
1/4 tsp. white pepper
Garnish: dill weed

In a microwave safe bowl, place cleaned and trimmed head of cauliflower. Sprinkle with 2 tablespoons of water, cover tightly with plastic food wrap, and microcook on high power for 6 to 8 minutes. Test cauliflower with a fork for desired doneness. Drain water from cauliflower. Meanwhile in a small glass measure, combine cheese, milk, mustard, and pepper. Microcook this mixture for 2 minutes on 70% power, stopping twice to stir. Pour cheese sauce over the steamed head of cauliflower and serve. Garnish with dill weed if desired.

93 calories, 4 gm. fat, 6 gm. protein, 7 gm. carbohydrate, 15 mg. cholesterol, 335 mg. sodium, 1.8 dietary fiber, 6 RE vitamin A, 52 mg. vitamin C, 0 vitamin E as alpha tocopherol

Food exchange
1 fat, 1 vegetable, 1/2 lean meat

Preparation time
10 minutes

Microcooking time
10 minutes

EGGPLANT PARMESAN

8 servings, 3/4 cup each

1 large eggplant
8-oz. can tomato sauce
4 oz. part-skim mozzarella cheese, shredded
1/3 cup Parmesan cheese

Peel eggplant and cut in half lengthwise. Then, cut each half into 1/2-inch thick slices. Spray an 11- by 7-inch microwave-safe casserole dish with nonstick cooking spray. Layer slices of eggplant with tomato sauce in the casserole dish. Sprinkle the top with mozzarella cheese and then Parmesan cheese. Cover and microcook on high power for 12 minutes. Serve as a topping over spaghetti.

72 calories, 3 gm. fat, 5 gm. protein, 5 gm. carbohydrate,
10 mg. cholesterol, 297 mg. sodium, 1.2 gm. dietary fiber,
25 RE vitamin A, 4 mg. vitamin C, 0 vitamin E as alpha tocopherol

Food exchange
1/2 lean meat, 1/2 fat, 1 vegetable

Preparation time
10 minutes

Cooking time
10 minutes

FRESH PEAS WITH SUGAR AND SPICE

8 servings, 1/2 cup each

4 cups fresh shelled peas
1/4 cup water
3 green onions, sliced fine, including tops
2 tsp. sugar
1/4 tsp. thyme
1 Tbsp. margarine

In a medium saucepan, combine fresh shelled peas with 1/4 cup water. Cover and cook over medium heat for 15 minutes. Drain peas and return to the saucepan. Add onion, sugar, thyme, and margarine. Cover and cook over low heat for another 5 minutes. Toss mixture to blend and serve.

97 calories, 1 gm. fat, 6 gm. protein, 16 gm. carbohydrate, 0 cholesterol, 25 mg. sodium, 2.6 gm. dietary fiber, 99 RE vitamin A, 49 mg. vitamin C, 0 vitamin E as alpha tocopherol

Food exchange
1 bread/starch, 1 vegetable

Preparation time
15 minutes

Cooking time
20 minutes

FRESH PEPPER STIR-FRY

Design your own pepper medley!

8 servings, 3/4 cup each

1 Tbsp. vegetable oil
1/2 tsp. garlic powder
2 green peppers, cut into rings with seeds removed
1 banana pepper, cut into rings with seeds
   removed
1 red pepper, cut into rings with seeds removed
1 yellow pepper, cut into rings with seeds removed
1 tsp. lemon pepper

In a large skillet, heat oil and garlic powder over medium heat for 2 minutes, stirring occasionally. Add pepper rings and continue to cook uncovered for 10 minutes, stirring frequently. Season with lemon pepper and serve. Makes a nice side dish with grilled beef or chicken.

52 calories, 1 gm. fat, 1 gm. protein, 9 gm. carbohydrate, 0 cholesterol, 2 mg. sodium, 1.1 gm. dietary fiber, 67 RE vitamin A, 179 mg. vitamin C, 0.8 mg. vitamin E as alpha tocopherol (using sunflower oil)

Food exchange
2 vegetable

Preparation time
15 minutes

Cooking time
12 minutes

FRUITY PARSNIPS

8 servings, 3/4 cup each

8 medium parsnips
1/4 cup water
2 Tbsp. brown sugar
1 Tbsp. cornstarch
Dash of salt
8-oz. can crushed pineapple in juice
1 tsp. shredded orange peel
1/2 cup orange juice
1/4 cup dark raisins
1 Tbsp. margarine

Peel and slice parsnips. Cook in a covered pan with 1/4 cup water over medium heat for 15 minutes, or until tender. Drain. In another small saucepan, blend brown sugar, cornstarch, and salt. Stir in pineapple, orange peel, and orange juice. Cook over medium heat, stirring constantly, until sauce is thickened. Fold in raisins and margarine. Place sliced parsnips in a serving bowl. Pour fruit sauce over them and fold gently. Serve with poultry or ham.

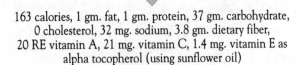

163 calories, 1 gm. fat, 1 gm. protein, 37 gm. carbohydrate,
0 cholesterol, 32 mg. sodium, 3.8 gm. dietary fiber,
20 RE vitamin A, 21 mg. vitamin C, 1.4 mg. vitamin E as
alpha tocopherol (using sunflower oil)

Food exchange
1 bread/starch, 1 fruit, 1 vegetable

Preparation time
15 minutes

Cooking time
20 minutes

GRANNY'S GREEN BEAN AND MUSHROOM CASSEROLE

Reduce the sodium and fat in an all-time favorite with this recipe.

8 servings, 1 cup each

2 16-oz. cans no-added-salt French-style green
  beans, well drained
8 oz. fresh mushrooms, sliced thin
13-oz. can reduced-fat, reduced-sodium cream of
  mushroom soup
1 tsp. reduced-sodium soy sauce
1 cup skim milk
1 cup onion-flavored croutons

Preheat oven to 375° F. Combine drained green beans and
mushrooms in a casserole dish. In a small mixing bowl,
blend soup, soy sauce, and skim milk. Fold the sauce into
beans. Garnish the top of the casserole with croutons.
Bake for 35 to 40 minutes.

110 calories, 4 gm. fat, 4 gm. protein, 14 gm. carbohydrate,
0 cholesterol, 432 mg. sodium (to reduce sodium, use unsalted bread
cubes as topping), 2.8 gm. dietary fiber, 58 RE vitamin A,
7 mg. vitamin C, 0 vitamin E as alpha tocopherol

Food exchange
2 vegetable, 1 fat

Preparation time
15 minutes

Baking time
40 minutes

GREEN BEANS PROVENCALE

8 servings, 3/4 cup each

16 oz. frozen green beans
1 Tbsp. margarine
1/4 tsp. garlic powder
1/4 cup finely chopped 97% fat-free ham
1/4 tsp. salt
1/8 tsp. black pepper
2 medium tomatoes, cut into wedges

Combine all ingredients in a large skillet. Cover and cook for 10 minutes over medium heat, stirring occasionally. Serve as a side dish with pasta or chicken.

38 calories, 1 gm. fat, 2 gm. protein, 6 gm. carbohydrate, 3 mg. cholesterol, 237 mg. sodium, 1 gm. dietary fiber, 49 RE vitamin A, 10 mg. vitamin C, 0 vitamin E as alpha tocopherol

Food exchange
2 vegetable

Preparation time
10 minutes

Cooking time
10 minutes

HARVARD BEETS

4 servings, 3/4 cup each

16-oz. can sliced beets
1 Tbsp. sugar
1 tsp. cornstarch
1/8 tsp. salt
2 Tbsp. vinegar
1 tsp. margarine
Garnish: Twisted slice of lemon

Drain beets and reserve 1/4 cup liquid. In a 1 1/2-quart microwave-safe bowl, mix sugar, cornstarch, and salt together. Stir in reserved liquid and vinegar. Microcook uncovered for 1 minute, stopping twice to stir. Stir in margarine and beets. Microcook an additional 2 minutes and serve. Garnish with a twisted lemon slice.

101 calories, 0 fat, 0 protein, 24 gm. carbohydrate, 0 cholesterol,
256 mg. sodium, 2 gm. dietary fiber, 8 RE vitamin A,
2 mg. vitamin C, 0 vitamin E as alpha tocopherol

Food exchange
1 bread/starch, 1 vegetable

Preparation time
10 minutes

Microcooking time
3 minutes

HAWAIIAN VEGETABLE KABOBS

8 servings, 1 cup each

20-oz. can unsweetened pineapple chunks, drained
2 large green peppers, cut into chunks
2 small white onions, quartered
8 fresh mushrooms
8 cherry tomatoes
1/2 cup reduced-sodium soy sauce
1 Tbsp. vegetable oil
1 Tbsp. brown sugar
1 tsp. ground ginger
1/2 tsp. garlic powder
1/2 tsp. dry mustard
1/4 tsp. pepper

Drain pineapple, reserving 1/4 cup juice. Place the pineapple and all of the vegetables in a bowl. In a shaker container, mix reserved pineapple juice with all remaining ingredients. Shake to blend well. Pour soy marinade over vegetables until grilling time. Arrange pineapple and vegetable chunks on 8 skewers. Grill for 20 minutes over low heat, basting frequently with marinade. These kabobs go well with fish, chicken, pork, or beef.

76 calories, 1 gm. fat, 2 gm. protein, 14 gm. carbohydrate, 0 cholesterol, 974 mg. sodium (to reduce sodium decrease soy sauce to 1/4 cup), 2 gm. dietary fiber, 37 RE vitamin A, 57 mg. vitamin C, 0.8 mg. vitamin E as alpha tocopherol (using sunflower oil)

Food exchange
1 vegetable, 1 fruit

Preparation time
15 minutes

Grilling time
20 minutes

KARLA'S SCALLOPED CELERY

8 servings, 3/4 cup each

1 bunch of celery, cleaned and diced into 1/2-inch
   pieces (save celery tops for garnish)
2 Tbsp. water
13-oz. can reduced-fat cream of chicken soup
1/4 cup skim milk
1 Tbsp. white wine Worcestershire sauce
Garnish: 1/4 cup toasted almonds

Place diced celery in a microwave-safe casserole dish, sprinkle with 2 tablespoons water and cover tightly. Microcook on high power for 6 to 8 minutes, until celery is fork-tender. Drain off liquid. Meanwhile, in a small mixing bowl, combine chicken soup, skim milk, and Worcestershire sauce. Microcook the soup mixture for 2 minutes, stopping twice to stir. Pour this mixture over drained celery and mix well. Microcook for 3 minutes longer to heat through. Garnish the top of the casserole with toasted almonds and chopped celery tops.

97 calories, 6 gm. fat, 3 gm. protein, 6 gm. carbohydrate, 4 mg. cholesterol, 459 mg. sodium, 0 dietary fiber, 32 RE vitamin A, 2 mg. vitamin C, 3.3 mg. vitamin E as alpha tocopherol

Food exchange
1 fat, 2 vegetable

Preparation time
10 minutes

Cooking time
10 minutes

NO-SALT SPICE BLEND FOR VEGETABLES

Recipe makes 1/2 cup
(Use about 1 tsp. for 4 servings of vegetables.)

1 tsp. basil
2 tsp. ground thyme
2 tsp. white pepper
2 tsp. garlic powder
2 Tbsp. paprika
2 Tbsp. onion powder
2 Tbsp. dry mustard
1 tsp. celery seed

Combine seasonings in a shaker container and use instead of salt with any hot vegetable.

This seasoning has negligible nutrient value and is used as a Free Food.

Preparation time
10 minutes

OKRA MEDLEY

8 servings, 1 cup each

4 strips of bacon, diced
16-oz. can whole kernel corn, drained well
10 oz. frozen okra
1 small yellow onion, chopped
1 Tbsp. chili powder
1 14-oz. can chopped tomatoes in juice

In a stockpot, cook bacon until crisp. Allow bacon to drain on a paper towel and discard the drippings. Add all remaining ingredients to the stockpot, and cook over high heat for 10 to 12 minutes, until onion is tender. Add the drained bacon and serve.

89 calories, 1 gm. fat, 3 gm. protein, 17 gm. carbohydrate,
2 mg. cholesterol, 163 mg. sodium, 2.6 gm. dietary fiber,
60 RE vitamin A, 14 mg. vitamin C,
0 vitamin E as alpha tocopherol

Food exchange
2 vegetable, 1/2 bread/starch

Preparation time
10 minutes

Baking time
20 minutes

RED CABBAGE WITH PINEAPPLE

8 servings, 1 cup each

6 cups shredded red cabbage
1 Tbsp. lemon juice
1/2 cup water
1 Tbsp. margarine
2 Tbsp. brown sugar
1 Tbsp. cornstarch
1/2 tsp. salt
2 Tbsp. vinegar
1 6-oz. can crushed pineapple, drained well
Reserved pineapple juice

In a large skillet, combine first three ingredients. Cook over medium heat for 10 minutes. Stir in margarine. In a shaker container, combine brown sugar, cornstarch, and salt. Shake to blend well. Add reserved pineapple juice and vinegar; shake until dry ingredients are dissolved. Add mixture to the cabbage and cook until thick. Stir in drained pineapple and heat through (2 more minutes). Makes a good side dish with pork.

89 calories, 1 gm. fat, 2 gm. protein, 17 gm. carbohydrate, 0 cholesterol, 167 mg. sodium, 2.6 gm. dietary fiber, 18 RE vitamin A, 99 mg. vitamin C, 1.3 mg. vitamin E as alpha tocopherol

Food exchange
1 vegetable, 1 fruit

Preparation time
10 minutes

Cooking time
17 minutes

SCALLOPED CABBAGE

8 servings, 1 cup each

1/4 cup water
1/2 tsp. salt
1 bag or 6 cups of shredded green cabbage
2 Tbsp. margarine
1/4 cup flour
1/4 tsp. black pepper
1 1/3 cups skim milk
4 oz. reduced-fat cheddar cheese, shredded
1/4 cup bread crumbs

In a 3-quart casserole dish, combine water, salt, and cabbage. Cover and microcook on high power for 8 minutes. Meanwhile, combine flour, pepper, and skim milk in a shaker container and shake until no lumps of flour remain. When cabbage is done, stir margarine and milk and flour mixture into the cabbage. Spread cheese and then bread crumbs over the top. Bake for 20 minutes at 375° F, or microcook on high power for 7 minutes.

161 calories, 6 gm. fat, 9 gm. protein, 20 gm. carbohydrate, 10 mg. cholesterol, 348 mg. sodium, 1 gm. dietary fiber, 104 RE vitamin A, 55 mg. vitamin C, 1.7 mg. vitamin E as alpha tocopherol

Food exchange
1 fat, 1 skim milk, 1 vegetable

Preparation time
10 minutes

Microcooking time + conventional cooking time
28 minutes

All microcook method
15 minutes

185

SKILLET EGGPLANT

8 servings, 3/4 cup each

1 large eggplant, peeled
1 Tbsp. cooking oil
1 slightly beaten egg or 1/4 cup liquid
  egg substitute
1 Tbsp. skim milk
1/2 cup bread crumbs
1 tsp. dry Italian blend seasoning mix

Cut eggplant in half lengthwise and then cut into 1/2-inch slices. Next, heat oil in large skillet over medium heat. In a shallow mixing bowl, combine egg with 1 Tbsp. milk. In a second shallow bowl, combine bread crumbs with Italian seasoning. Dip slices of eggplant in egg mixture and then in bread crumbs. Cook in a large skillet for 3 minutes on each side, until evenly browned.

57 calories, 2 gm. fat, 1 gm. protein, 8 gm. carbohydrate,
0 cholesterol, 67 mg. sodium, 1.2 gm. dietary fiber,
4 RE vitamin A, 0 vitamin C, 0.8 mg. vitamin E as
alpha tocopherol (using sunflower oil)

Food exchange
1 vegetable, 1/2 fat

Preparation time
15 minutes

Cooking time
12 minutes

SPICY GREEN BEAN AND TOMATO MEDLEY

8 servings, 1 cup each

1 large onion, chopped fine
4 ribs of celery, chopped fine
2 large carrots, cut into coins
1 large green pepper, cut into strips
14-oz. can chunky tomatoes, including juice
1 Tbsp. oil
1/4 tsp. black pepper
1 Tbsp. sugar
1/4 tsp. salt
2 Tbsp. minute tapioca
16-oz. can no-added-salt green beans, drained well

Combine all ingredients except the green beans in a 3-quart casserole dish. Stir to mix. Cover and bake for 1 hour at 375 ° F; or microcook on high power for 20 minutes, stirring three times during the 20-minute cooking time. Stir in the green beans 5 minutes before the end of the cooking time with either method.

83 calories, 2 gm. fat, 2 gm. protein, 16 gm. carbohydrate,
0 cholesterol, 357 mg. sodium, 3 gm. dietary fiber,
579 RE vitamin A, 41 mg. vitamin C, 0.8 mg. vitamin E as
alpha tocopherol (using sunflower oil)

Food exchange
2 vegetable, 1/2 fat

Preparation time
15 minutes

Baking time
1 hour

Microcooking time
20 minutes

SWEET AND SOUR KALE

8 servings, 1 cup each

1 lb. fresh kale
4 slices bacon, diced
2 Tbsp. flour
1 1/2 cup hot water
2 Tbsp. sugar
2 Tbsp. vinegar
1/4 tsp. black pepper

Cut roots of the kale and remove any brown leaves. Cut stems and leaves into small pieces. Heat 5 to 6 quarts of water to boiling in a large kettle. Add greens and cook until tender, about 1 hour. Meanwhile, in a skillet, cook diced bacon until crisp. Drain bacon on a paper towel and discard drippings. In a shaker container, mix flour, water, sugar, vinegar, and black pepper until no lumps remain. Pour this mixture in the skillet and cook over medium heat for 4 to 6 minutes until thick, stirring frequently. When greens are tender, drain well and transfer to a large bowl. Pour the cooked sauce over the greens, fold in bacon pieces, and serve.

66 calories, 1 gm. fat, 3 gm. protein, 12 gm. carbohydrate, 2 mg. cholesterol, 62 mg. sodium, 1.2 gm. dietary fiber, 504 RE vitamin A, 68 mg. vitamin C, 0 vitamin E as alpha tocopherol

Food exchange
1 vegetable, 1/2 bread/starch

Preparation time
15 minutes

Cooking time
1 hour

SWEET AND SOUR RED CABBAGE

8 servings, 1 cup each

1 medium red cabbage, shredded
1 small onion, sliced
2 Tbsp. lemon juice
4 slices bacon, diced
1/4 cup brown sugar
2 Tbsp. flour
1/2 cup water
1/4 cup vinegar
1/2 tsp. salt
1/8 tsp. black pepper

In a casserole dish, combine shredded cabbage with sliced onion and lemon juice. Cover and microcook for 8 minutes. Meanwhile, in a small skillet, fry diced bacon until crisp. Discard drippings. Remove bacon and allow to drain on a paper towel. In the same skillet, combine brown sugar, flour, water, vinegar, salt, and pepper. Whisk mixture smooth; then cook over medium heat until thick, about 5 minutes. Pour sauce over cooked cabbage. Stir to mix. Stir in diced bacon and microcook on high power 2 minutes longer. Makes a good side dish with roast pork.

81 calories, 1 gm. fat, 2 gm. protein, 16 gm. carbohydrate, 2 mg. cholesterol, 16 mg. sodium, 2.6 dietary fiber, 2 RE vitamin A, 50 mg. vitamin C, 0 vitamin E as alpha tocopherol

Food exchange
1 bread/starch

Preparation time
10 minutes

Microcooking time
10 minutes

SWEET AND TANGY CARROTS IN THE MICROWAVE

8 servings, 3/4 cup each

2 lb. fresh carrots
1/4 cup fresh lemon juice
1/4 cup firmly-packed brown sugar
1/3 cup raisins
1 Tbsp. margarine

Choose firm, clean, well-shaped bright orange carrots.
Scrub, peel, and slice into coins in a 2-quart microwave-safe
dish. Sprinkle with lemon juice, brown sugar, and raisins.
Cover and microcook on high power for 8 to 10 minutes
until carrots are tender-crisp. Dot with margarine and serve.

73 calories, 1 gm. fat, 4 gm. protein, 12 gm. carbohydrate, 0 cholesterol, 33 mg. sodium, 3 gm. dietary fiber, 2872 RE vitamin A,
6 mg. vitamin C, 0 vitamin E as alpha tocopherol

Food exchange
1 vegetable, 1/2 fruit

Preparation time
10 minutes

Microcooking time
10 minutes

VEGETABLE KABOBS ON THE GRILL

4 servings, 1 cup each

1 medium zucchini or yellow squash
2 small onions
1 Tbsp. nonfat Italian salad dressing
2 Tbsp. Parmesan cheese
Fresh ground pepper

Halve the zucchini lengthwise and cut into 1-inch chunks.
Peel and quarter the onions. Alternate zucchini and onion
on 4 skewers. Arrange the skewers on a large sheet of
waxed paper. Sprinkle evenly with salad dressing, cheese,
and pepper. Rotate skewers during preparation to evenly
coat. Broil or grill vegetables 2 inches from the heat source
for 8 minutes, turning twice during cooking.

36 calories, 0 fat, 2 gm. protein, 5 gm. carbohydrate,
2 mg. cholesterol, 50 mg. sodium, 1.6 gm. dietary fiber, 38 RE
vitamin A, 11 mg. vitamin C, 0 vitamin E as alpha tocopherol

Food exchange
1 vegetable

Preparation time
10 minutes

Broiling time
8 minutes

WESTERN YELLOW SQUASH

4 servings, 1 cup each

2 medium yellow squash
1/2 cup reduced-calorie western-style French
   dressing
1/2 tsp. celery seed

Quarter the squash lengthwise to form 8 spears. Rub the cut surfaces of the squash with salad dressing. Sprinkle with celery seed. Lay the spears on the grill and broil 2 inches from the heat source for 8 minutes, turning twice during cooking.

64 calories, 0 fat, 2 gm. protein, 13 gm. carbohydrate, 0 cholesterol,
3 mg. sodium, 2.4 gm. dietary fiber, 45 RE vitamin A,
33 mg. vitamin C, 1.1 mg. vitamin E as alpha tocopherol
(from dressing)

Food exchange
1 vegetable, 1/2 fruit

Preparation time
10 minutes

Broiling time
8 minutes

ZUCCHINI-STUFFED TOMATO

4 servings, 1 tomato each

4 large, firm tomatoes
2 medium zucchini, grated
1 small onion, chopped fine
1 cup reduced-fat Swiss cheese
1/4 tsp. salt
1/4 tsp. pepper
1/2 tsp. basil

Preheat oven to 375° F. Wash tomatoes, and cut off the tops. Scoop out pulp and reserve for use in a vegetable soup or vegetable juice cocktail. In a mixing bowl, combine all remaining ingredients. Stuff zucchini and cheese mixture into the tomato shells. Bake for 10 minutes. Do not overbake, as tomato shells will not retain their shape. Serve hot. Makes a nice side dish with grilled hamburgers.

121 calories, 5 gm. fat, 12 gm. protein, 7 gm. carbohydrate, 207 mg. cholesterol, 140 mg. sodium, 2.4 gm. dietary fiber, 273 RE vitamin A, 44 mg. vitamin C, 1.1 mg. vitamin E as alpha tocopherol

Food exchange
1 lean meat, 2 vegetable, 1/2 fat

Preparation time
15 minutes

Baking time
10 minutes

ENTREES

BECKY'S REUNION POTATOES

16 servings, 1 cup each

1 lb. lean ground beef
1-oz. envelope taco seasoning mix
24-oz. bag frozen hash browns with pepper and
    onion, thawed
13-oz. can cream of cheddar cheese soup
4-oz. can green chilies, drained
1 cup skim milk
Garnish: 1/2 cup chunky salsa

Preheat oven to 375° F. Brown ground beef in a skillet and
drain well. If the meat appears fatty, place it in a colander
over a bowl and rinse it with 1 cup of boiling water; drain
5 minutes longer. Place drained meat in a 9- by 13-inch
baking pan. Sprinkle taco seasoning over the browned
meat. Sprinkle hash-brown potatoes over the taco seasoning. In a mixing bowl, mix cheese soup, green chilies, and
skim milk until smooth. Pour over potatoes. Bake for 1
hour until potatoes are tender. Garnish the casserole with
chunky salsa before serving.

181 calories, 7 gm. fat, 10 gm. protein, 18 gm. carbohydrate, 722
mg. sodium (to reduce sodium use only half of the taco seasoning
mix), 0.8 gm.dietary fiber, 109 RE vitamin A, 16 mg. vitamin C,
0 vitamin E as alpha tocopherol

Food exchange
1 bread/starch, 1 lean meat, 1 fat

Preparation time
20 minutes

Baking time
1 hour

CALICO BEAN CASSEROLE

16 servings, 2/3 cup each

1/4 lb. Canadian bacon, cut into 1/2-inch chunks
1 medium onion, chopped fine
28-oz. can pork and beans with tomato sauce
15-oz. can butter beans, drained
15-oz. can pinto beans, drained
1/4 cup brown sugar
1/2 cup catsup
2 Tbsp. vinegar
1 tsp. dry mustard
1/4 cup molasses

Combine all ingredients in a crockpot and cook on low for
4 to 6 hours. If you are in a hurry, this can be heated in the
microwave oven. To do so, mix all ingredients in a 3-quart
casserole dish, cover and microcook on 70% power for 18
to 20 minutes, stirring twice during cooking.

188 calories, 3 gm. fat, 9 gm. protein, 32 gm. carbohydrate, 7 mg.
cholesterol, 431 mg. sodium, 5.7 gm. dietary fiber, 7 RE vitamin A,
4 mg. vitamin C, 0 vitamin E as alpha tocopherol

Food exchange
1 1/2 bread/starch, 1 lean meat

Preparation time
10 minutes

Crockpot cooking time
4 to 6 hours

Microcooking time
20 minutes

CINDY'S UNBEATABLE PRESSURE-COOKER BEANS

16 servings, 1 cup each

2 lb. small red beans, dry
2 tsp. baking soda
1/2 lb. bacon, diced, cooked crisp, and drained well
1/2 cup molasses
1 cup brown sugar
1 tsp. dry mustard
1 tsp. ginger
46 oz. tomato juice

Place all ingredients in a pressure cooker. Add water to fill the cooker within 2 inches of the top. Place the pressure control on the top after setting the weight to 15 pounds of pressure. Turn heat on low, increase to medium low and as soon as the pressure control begins to jiggle, return the heat to low. Cook for 40 minutes. Turn off and allow cooker to cool for 30 minutes. Remove cover carefully and add 2 cups of water. Stir to mix and serve.

254 calories, 7 gm. fat, 13 gm. protein, 35 gm. carbohydrate, 12 mg. cholesterol, 456 mg. sodium, 5.2 gm.dietary fiber, 45 RE vitamin A, 12 mg. vitamin C, 1.1 mg. vitamin E as alpha tocopherol

Food exchange
1/2 fruit, 1 lean meat, 2 bread/starch

Preparation time
15 minutes

Cooking time
40 minutes

Cooling time
30 minutes

CRUNCHY WILD RICE SALAD

A great prescription for leftover meat!

8 servings, 1 cup each

1 cup uncooked brown and wild rice blend
1/4 tsp. seasoned salt
2 cups diced cooked meat of choice (try chicken, ham, or roast pork)
1 1/2 cup green grapes, halved
8-oz. can sliced water chestnuts, well drained
2 ribs celery, sliced thin
3/4 cup reduced-fat mayonnaise
1 Tbsp. lemon juice
1 tsp. sugar

Cook rice according to package directions. Fluff cooked rice with a fork, and cool to room temperature. In a large salad bowl, combine cooled rice with salt, meat, grapes, water chestnuts, and celery. In a small mixing bowl, blend mayonnaise, lemon juice, and sugar. Fold dressing into rice mixture and serve or chill until serving time.

229 calories, 9 gm. fat, 18 gm. protein, 17 gm. carbohydrate, 55 mg. cholesterol, 261 mg. sodium, 0 dietary fiber, 8 RE vitamin A, 3 mg. vitamin C, 0 vitamin E as alpha tocopherol

Food exchange
1 vegetable, 2 lean meat, 1 bread/starch

Preparation time
15 minutes

Cooking time
15 minutes

CHICKEN AND VEGETABLE SALAD

8 servings, 3/4 cup each plus 1 cup greens

1 Tbsp. vegetable oil
4 whole chicken breasts, skinned, boned, and cut
   into 1/2-inch cubes
5 large carrots, sliced thin
1/4 tsp. ground ginger
1 bunch green onions, diced
1 large red pepper, diced
1 large yellow pepper, diced
1/4 cup reduced-sodium soy sauce
2 Tbsp. cider vinegar
2 tsp. brown sugar
1 Tbsp. vegetable oil
8 cups fresh greens
Garnish: 1/2 cup chow mein noodles

In a large skillet, saute chicken with carrots and ginger in oil over medium heat for 8 to 10 minutes until chicken is cooked through. Put the mixture in a salad bowl. Meanwhile, dice green onions and peppers; mix with the carrots and chicken. In a shaker container, mix soy sauce, vinegar, brown sugar, and vegetable oil until well-blended. Add dressing to chicken and vegetables and blend. Arrange the greens on 8 plates. Divide chicken salad among the 8 plates. Garnish with chow mein noodles and serve.

273 calories, 8 gm. fat, 32 gm. protein, 19 gm. carbohydrate, 73 mg. cholesterol, 558 mg. sodium (to reduce sodium, use just 2 Tbsp. soy sauce), 2.4 gm. dietary fiber, 1885 RE vitamin A, 167 mg. vitamin C, 1.6 mg. vitamin E as alpha tocopherol (using sunflower oil)

Food exchange
4 lean meat, 1/2 bread/starch, 1 vegetable

Preparation time
20 minutes

Cooking time
10 minutes

HERBED ORZO WITH RICE AND VEGETABLES

12 servings, 1 cup each

1 cup dry orzo
1 cup dry brown rice
3 qt. water
20-oz. pkg. frozen San Francisco blend vegetables
    (broccoli, red and green peppers, French-style
    green beans, and onions)
1 Tbsp. margarine
1 tsp. dried basil
1 tsp. dried oregano
1 tsp. ground thyme
1 tsp. salt
1 tsp. pepper
1/2 cup grated Parmesan cheese

In a large stockpot, combine orzo and rice with 3 quarts of water. Bring to a boil, then reduce heat to simmer and cook for 20 minutes. Drain well. Meanwhile, place vegetables in a microwave-safe casserole dish, cover, and microcook on high power for 6 minutes. Place rice and orzo in a shallow casserole dish for serving; stir in margarine, basil, oregano, thyme, salt, and pepper. Top with steamed vegetables, and garnish with Parmesan cheese.

184 calories, 3 gm. fat, 6 gm. protein, 33 gm. carbohydrate, 2 mg. cholesterol, 260 mg. sodium, 1 gm. dietary fiber, 256 RE vitamin A, 1 mg. vitamin C, 0 vitamin E as alpha tocopherol

Food exchange
2 bread/starch, 1 vegetable

Preparation time
10 minutes

Cooking time
20 minutes

HOT WEATHER SPAGHETTI

8 servings, 1 cup each

4 large ripe tomatoes
1 Tbsp. vegetable oil
2 Tbsp. red wine vinegar
1/4 tsp. salt
1/8 tsp. pepper
3 Tbsp. chopped green onions
1 tsp. dried basil
1 tsp. dried oregano
1/4 tsp. fennel
3 qt. water
1/8 tsp. salt
8 oz. spaghetti

Peel tomatoes and chop or process in a food processor until chunky. In a mixing bowl, combine chopped tomatoes with all remaining ingredients except the salt and spaghetti. Meanwhile, bring 3 quarts of water to a boil; add salt and spaghetti. Boil for 8 minutes, drain, and rinse with cold water. Serve spaghetti with cold tomato dressing.

135 calories, 2 gm. fat, 4 gm. protein, 24 gm. carbohydrate, 0 cholesterol, 168 mg. sodium, 1 gm. dietary fiber, 40 RE vitamin A, 12 mg. vitamin C, 0.8 mg. vitamin E as alpha tocopherol (using sunflower oil)

Food exchange
1 vegetable, 1 1/2 bread/starch

Preparation time
15 minutes

Cooking time
8 minutes

MONTEREY SKILLET VEGETABLES

This is a version of a recipe passed to me by a fellow dietitian-author and mentor, Mabel Caviani.

8 servings, 1 cup each

8 small zucchini
1 Tbsp. vegetable oil
1 large yellow onion, coarsely chopped
1 4-oz. can diced green chilies
1 14-oz. can diced tomatoes in juice
1 8-oz. can whole kernel corn, drained well
1/2 tsp. garlic powder
1/2 tsp. salt
1/8 tsp. pepper
8 oz. reduced-fat Monterey Jack cheese, shredded
Garnish: paprika

Wash zucchini and trim ends. Cut crosswise into 1/4-inch slices and set aside. In a large skillet, saute onions with green chilies for 2 minutes. Add tomatoes and continue cooking 2 minutes. Add zucchini and corn and cook over medium heat uncovered for 10 minutes. Stir in garlic powder, salt, and pepper and continue cooking until heated through and most of the liquid has been reduced. Sprinkle the vegetables with cheese and then sprinkle the cheese with paprika. Serve when the cheese is melted. This makes a wonderful light supper with a crusty roll and fresh fruit. Fresh tomatoes and corn can be used instead of the canned varieties.

162 calories, 7 gm. fat, 12 gm. protein, 15 gm. carbohydrate, 20 mg. cholesterol, 482 mg. sodium, 2.8 gm. dietary fiber, 145 RE vitamin A, 27 mg. vitamin C, 0.8 mg. vitamin E as alpha tocopherol (using sunflower oil)

Food exchange
1 vegetable, 1 lean meat, 1 bread/starch

Preparation time
15 minutes

Cooking time
20 minutes

NORMANDY ENDIVE SUPREME

For Dr. Wayne and Sharon Kelly, our traveling companions through Normandy in the spring of 1994.

8 servings, 3 cups each

> 2 large Belgian endive, cleaned and leaves torn
> from stem
> 4 large carrots, grated
> 8 radishes, sliced
> 8 oz. bean sprouts
> 1 rib celery, chopped
> 1 small red onion, chopped
> 8 oz. reduced-fat mozzarella cheese, shredded
> 8 oz. Canadian bacon, diced
> *Dressing:* Choose your own reduced-fat herb and
> vinegar dressing

Layer salad ingredients on dinner plates in order listed. Serve with reduced-fat herb and vinegar dressing and hot French bread.

195 calories, 8 gm. fat, 21 gm. protein, 12 gm. carbohydrate, 36 mg. cholesterol, 811 mg. sodium (to reduce sodium, substitute lean cooked pork for bacon), 3.8 gm. dietary fiber, 2234 RE vitamin A, 85 mg. vitamin C, 0 vitamin E as alpha tocopherol

Food exchange
2 lean meat, 3 vegetable

Preparation time
20 minutes

PEACHES AND PORK

8 servings, 4 oz. pork plus 1/2 cup peaches each

2 lb. pork tenderloin, trimmed well
1/4 tsp. salt
1/4 tsp. black pepper
2 tsp. vegetable oil
4 fresh peaches, halved, pitted, and cut into
   wedges
1 large red pepper, seeded and chopped into strips
3 large green onions, diced
1/2 tsp. ground ginger
2 tsp. soy sauce

Cut pork into thin slices and sprinkle with salt and pepper.
Heat oil in a large skillet over medium heat. Add pork and
cook for 3 minutes on each side until browned. Remove
browned pork to a platter. Add peaches, red pepper, and
green onions to the skillet and cook over medium heat for
4 minutes. Return browned pork to the skillet, sprinkle
with ginger and soy sauce, and cover the skillet. Reduce
heat to medium-low and cook for 5 minutes, until pork is
cooked through. Serve over brown rice.

262 calories, 12 gm. fat, 28 gm. protein, 12 gm. carbohydrate,
76 mg. cholesterol, 224 mg. sodium, 2.5 gm. dietary fiber, 64 RE
vitamin A, 71 mg. vitamin C, 0 vitamin E as alpha tocopherol

Food exchange
4 lean meat, 1/2 fruit

Preparation time
20 minutes

PESTO FOR VEGETABLES AND PASTA

6 servings, 2 tablespoons each

1 cup fresh basil leaves
1 Tbsp. olive oil
1 garlic clove, minced
1/4 cup Parmesan cheese
1 Tbsp. chopped pine nuts or walnuts

Combine fresh basil with olive oil in a blender or food processor. Process to a smooth paste. Combine with minced garlic, Parmesan cheese, and chopped nuts. Serve as a topping to steamed vegetables or pasta. This keeps in the refrigerator for 5 days.

47 calories, 4 gm. fat, 1 gm. protein, 0 carbohydrate, 2 mg. cholesterol, 58 mg. sodium, 0 dietary fiber, 0 RE vitamin A, 0 vitamin C, 0 vitamin E as alpha tocopherol

Food exchange
1 fat

Preparation time
15 minutes

POTATO SALAD WITH CHICKEN

8 servings, 1 1/2 cup each

6 large red-skinned potatoes, scrubbed and cut
  into 1/2-inch chunks
8 cherry tomatoes
3 green onions
2 chicken breasts
1/4 cup lemon juice
2 Tbsp. vegetable oil
1/4 cup chopped fresh parsley
1/2 tsp. garlic powder
1 tsp. salt
1 tsp. paprika
1 tsp. cumin

Place potato chunks in a large saucepan, cover with 3
inches of boiling water, and simmer over medium heat for
15 minutes. Drain. Meanwhile, wash tomatoes and cut in
half; dice onions. In a small skillet, cook chicken breast
until done and then dice. In a shaker container, mix
remaining ingredients for dressing. At serving time, toss
potatoes, onions, tomatoes, and diced chicken with dressing. Serve with toasted pita bread.

167 calories, 4 gm. fat, 7 gm. protein, 26 gm. carbohydrate, 11 mg.
cholesterol, 289 mg. sodium, 3.4 gm. dietary fiber, 56 RE vitamin A,
32 mg. vitamin C, 1.6 mg. vitamin E as alpha tocopherol
(using sunflower oil)

Food exchange
1 lean meat, 1 vegetable, 1 bread/starch

Preparation time
30 minutes

STUFF ZUCCHINI THREE WAYS

8 servings, 1 zucchini each

For all three stuffings, start with:

8 medium zucchini
1 tsp. oil
1/2 tsp. garlic powder
1 medium onion, chopped fine

RICE AND BEANS STUFFING:

16-oz. can pinto beans, well drained
1 cup instant rice
1 cup chicken broth
2 Tbsp. chopped fresh parsley
Topping: 4 oz. part-skim mozzarella cheese, shredded
2 Tbsp. chopped green chilies

160 calories, 4 gm. fat, 10 gm. protein, 23 gm. carbohydrate,
7 mg. cholesterol, 525 mg. sodium, 5.8 gm. dietary fiber, 109 RE
vitamin A, 36 mg. vitamin C, 0 vitamin E as alpha tocopherol

Food exchange
1 lean meat, 1 1/2 bread/starch

PIZZA STUFFING:

1 1/2 cups dry macaroni
1 1/2 cups spaghetti sauce
1 cup water
1 tsp. basil
1 tsp. oregano
Topping: 1/2 cup Parmesan cheese

260 calories, 3 gm. fat, 13 gm. protein, 47 gm. carbohydrate,
3 mg. cholesterol, 117 mg. sodium, 3.2 gm. dietary fiber, 326 RE
vitamin A, 26 mg. vitamin C, 0 vitamin E as alpha tocopherol

Food exchange
2 bread/starch, 1 lean meat, 2 vegetable

CALIFORNIA VEGGIE STUFFING:

20-oz. pkg. California Blend frozen vegetables
13-oz. can reduced-fat cream of mushroom soup
Topping: 4 oz. reduced-fat cheddar cheese, shredded

168 calories, 6 gm. fat, 10 gm. protein, 21 gm. carbohydrate,
10 mg. cholesterol, 451 mg. sodium, 1.2 gm. dietary fiber, 409 RE
vitamin A, 24 mg. vitamin C, 0 vitamin E as alpha tocopherol

Food exchange
1 lean meat, 1 bread/starch, 1 vegetable

Cut zucchini in half lengthwise and scoop out the pulp,
leaving the shells 1/4 inch thick. Reserve the shells. Heat
oil in a medium skillet over high heat. Chop zucchini pulp
and add to pre-heated skillet along with onion and garlic.
Cook for 3 minutes. Stir in ingredients for stuffing and
cook over medium heat for 8 more minutes. Stuff zucchini
shells and place stuffed shells into an 11- by 8-inch
microwave-safe baking dish. Sprinkle shells with toppings.
Cover and microwave on high power for 6 to 8 minutes
until zucchini shells are tender-crisp.

Preparation time
15 minutes

Cooking time
20 minutes

STUFFED PEPPERS THREE WAYS

8 servings, 1 pepper each

8 large, firm green peppers

GARDEN WAY:

16-oz. can whole kernel corn, well drained
1 small onion, finely diced
13-oz. can tomato soup
1 Tbsp. chili powder
Topping: 4 oz. reduced-fat cheddar cheese, shredded

192 calories, 4 gm. fat, 8 gm. protein, 31 gm. carbohydrate,
10 mg. cholesterol, 379 mg. sodium, 2.6 gm. dietary fiber, 205 RE
vitamin A, 222 mg. vitamin C, 0 vitamin E as alpha tocopherol

Food exchange
1 1/2 bread/starch, 2 vegetable, 1/2 lean meat

MEXICALI WAY:

2 cup cooked rice (follow pkg. directions)
16-oz. can pinto beans, well drained
1 cup mild salsa
Topping: 4 oz. reduced-fat Monterey jack cheese,
shredded

195 calories, 3 gm. fat, 10 gm. protein, 34 gm. carbohydrate, 10 mg. cholesterol, 655 mg. sodium, 4.8 gm. dietary fiber, 214 RE vitamin A, 206 mg. vitamin C, 0 vitamin E as alpha tocopherol

Food exchange
1 lean meat, 1 vegetable, 1 1/2 bread/starch

BEEF AND BARLEY WAY:

2 cups cooked barley (follow pkg. directions)
3 ribs celery, chopped fine
8-oz. can sliced mushrooms, well drained
13-oz. can beefy mushroom soup
Topping: minced fresh parsley

160 calories, 2 gm. fat, 11 gm. protein, 27 gm. carbohydrate, 2 mg. cholesterol, 24 mg. sodium, 8 gm. dietary fiber, 146 RE vitamin A, 204 mg. vitamin C, 0 vitamin E as alpha tocopherol

Food exchange
1 lean meat, 1 vegetable, 1 bread/starch

Preheat oven to 375° F. Remove tops and seeds from peppers. Mix ingredients for stuffing in a mixing bowl. Carefully stuff peppers and sprinkle with topping. Place on a baking sheet and bake for 45 minutes. Peppers should be tender-crisp, yet retain their shape for serving.

Preparation time
15 minutes

Baking time
45 minutes

VEGGIE BURRITOS THREE WAYS

8 servings, 1 burrito each

8 large flour tortillas

CAULIFLOWER STUFFING:

20-oz. pkg. frozen cauliflower, thawed
2 large carrots, scrubbed and grated
1/2 cup reduced-fat ricotta cheese
4 oz. reduced-fat cheddar cheese, shredded

196 calories, 6 gm. fat, 10 gm. protein, 25 gm. carbohydrate, 14 mg.
cholesterol, 315 mg. sodium, 2.2 gm. dietary fiber, 555 RE
vitamin A, 23 mg. vitamin C, 0 vitamin E as alpha tocopherol

Food exchange
1 bread/starch, 1 lean meat, 2 vegetable

BACON AND BEAN STUFFING:

20-oz. can pork and beans, pork fat cube removed
8 strips bacon, cooked, drained, and diced
1/4 cup molasses
2 Tbsp. prepared mustard

257 calories, 6 gm. fat, 9 gm. protein, 42 gm. carbohydrate, 6 mg.
cholesterol, 647 mg. sodium, 4 gm. dietary fiber, 13 RE vitamin A,
2 mg. vitamin C, 0 vitamin E as alpha tocopherol

Food exchange
1 fat, 2 bread/starch, 2 vegetable

STIR-FRY VEGGIE STUFFING:

20-oz. pkg. stir-fry blend frozen vegetables, thawed
13-oz. can reduced-fat cream of mushroom soup
1/4 cup teriyaki sauce

212 calories, 6 gm. fat, 5 gm. protein, 33 gm. carbohydrate,
0 cholesterol, 754 mg. sodium (to reduce sodium, use reduced-sodium teriyaki sauce), 2 gm. dietary fiber, 302 RE vitamin A,
2 mg. vitamin C, 0 vitamin E as alpha tocopherol

Food exchange
2 vegetable, 1 1/2 bread/starch, 1 fat

Preheat oven to 375° F. Combine ingredients for stuffing in a large mixing bowl. Lay tortillas out flat and divide stuffing among the eight. Spoon the stuffing toward one side of the tortilla, then start rolling tortilla on that side, folding outside edge over on the bottom. Place burritos on a baking sheet, and bake for 30 minutes or until heated through.

Preparation time
15 minutes

Cooking time
30 minutes

VEGETABLE HASH WITH BACON

8 servings, 1 cup each

2 Tbsp. vegetable oil
6 red-skinned potatoes, washed, halved, and sliced
very thin
8 oz. Canadian bacon, diced
1 green pepper, diced
1 yellow onion, diced
1 tsp. salt
1/2 tsp. fresh ground pepper

In a large skillet, heat oil over medium heat. Add thin-sliced potatoes and cook for 15 to 18 minutes, covered. Add all remaining ingredients. Cover again and cook for 5 more minutes. Serve with light rye bread.

259 calories, 6 gm. fat, 11 gm. protein, 41 gm. carbohydrate,
16 mg. cholesterol, 717 mg. sodium (to reduce sodium, substitute
lean cooked pork for bacon), 2.6 gm. dietary fiber,
18 RE vitamin A, 56 mg. vitamin C, 1.6 mg. vitamin E as
alpha tocopherol (using sunflower oil)

Food exchange
2 vegetable, 2 bread/starch, 1 lean meat

Preparation time
15 minutes

Cooking time
25 minutes

VEGETARIAN CHILI IN THE CROCKPOT

8 servings, 1 cup each

3 Tbsp. chili powder
1 tsp. cumin
1/4 tsp. salt
1/2 tsp. oregano
1/2 tsp. pepper
2 Tbsp. tomato paste
14-oz. can whole tomatoes
1/2 tsp. garlic powder
2 large onions, finely chopped
16-oz. pkg. frozen mixed vegetables
2 15-oz. cans black beans, rinsed and drained
1 large jalapeno pepper, seeded and minced
    (*optional*)

Place all ingredients in a crockpot or slow cooker and cook
on low for 8 to 10 hours or on high for 4 to 6 hours.

157 calories, 1 gm. fat, 6 gm. protein, 31 gm. carbohydrate,
8 mg. cholesterol, 179 mg. sodium, 8.2 mg. dietary fiber, 293 RE
vitamin A, 15 mg. vitamin C, 0 vitamin E as alpha tocopherol

Food exchange
1 1/2 bread/starch, 2 vegetable

Preparation time
15 minutes

Slow cooker time:
4 to 6 hours on high heat; 8 to 10 hours on low heat

VEGETARIAN PIZZA

8 servings, 1 slice each

1 loaf frozen bread dough
2 cups spaghetti sauce of choice
3 cups fresh veggies of choice (diced onion and green pepper, sliced mushrooms, pineapple tidbits, grated carrots, and whole pea pods are good choices)
8 oz. reduced-fat mozzarella cheese, shredded
1/4 cup Parmesan cheese

Thaw bread dough in the refrigerator or at room temperature until it is easy to work with. Roll out bread dough on a 12-inch pizza pan sprayed with nonstick cooking spray. Preheat oven to 425° F. Place pizza pan with bread dough crust in the oven and bake for 10 minutes. Remove from oven, spread with sauce, choice of vegetables, and cheeses. Return to oven and bake for 15 more minutes. Veggies should be tender-crisp.

296 calories, 10 gm. fat, 14 gm. protein, 37 gm. carbohydrate, 21 mg. cholesterol, 777 mg. sodium, 1.2 gm. dietary fiber, 155 RE vitamin A, 37 mg. vitamin C, 0 vitamin E as alpha tocopherol

Food exchange
1 lean meat, 2 bread/starch, 1 vegetable, 1 fat

Preparation time
15 minutes

Baking time
25 minutes

VEGGIE BURGERS REINVENTED

8 servings, 1 burger each

2 lb. lean ground beef, pork, or turkey

Form 8 patties from ground meat and grill 2 inches from medium flame for 6 minutes on each side. Serve with rolls or breads and toppings from choices below.

BOSTON VARIETY:

16 slices Boston brown bread
1 cup baked beans, heated
4 bacon strips, cooked, drained, and diced
1/4 cup chili sauce

420 calories, 10 gm. fat, 36 gm. protein, 46 gm. carbohydrate, 98 mg. cholesterol, 890 mg. sodium (to reduce sodium, use just 2 tablespoons chili sauce), 5 gm. dietary fiber, 20 RE vitamin A, 2 mg. vitamin C, 0 vitamin E as alpha tocopherol

Food exchange
4 lean meat, 2 bread/starch, 2 vegetable

ENGLISH VARIETY:

8 toasted English muffins
1 large red onion, cut into rings
8 leaves romaine lettuce
1/2 cup chutney

376 calories, 11 gm.fat, 37 gm.protein, 33 gm.carbohydrate, 114 mg. cholesterol, 414 mg. sodium, 2 gm.dietary fiber, 73 RE vitamin A, 8 mg. vitamin C, 0 vitamin E as alpha tocopherol

Food exchange
4 lean meat, 2 bread/starch

SPA VARIETY:

8 whole-grain buns
1 cup green pea pods
1 cup chopped broccoli
1 cup bean sprouts

304 calories, 8 gm. fat, 34 gm. protein, 22 gm. carbohydrate, 94 mg. cholesterol, 284 mg. sodium, 5.2 gm. dietary fiber, 47 RE vitamin A, 43 mg. vitamin C, 0 vitamin E as alpha tocopherol

Food exchange
4 lean meat, 1 bread/starch

MIDWEST VARIETY:

8 bakery rolls
8 leaves iceberg lettuce
8 slices fresh tomato
1/2 cup dill pickle chips
1/4 cup chopped white onion

340 calories, 8 gm. fat, 34 gm. protein, 32 gm. carbohydrate, 94 mg. cholesterol, 573 mg. sodium, 1.6 gm. dietary fiber, 21 RE vitamin A, 4 mg. vitamin C, 0 vitamin E as alpha tocopherol

Food exchange
4 lean meat, 1 1/2 bread/starch

GERMAN VARIETY:

16 slices rye bread
1 cup drained sauerkraut
1/2 cup non-fat sour cream

354 calories, 8 gm. fat, 35 gm. protein, 33 gm. carbohydrate, 94 mg.
cholesterol, 800 mg. sodium, 3.8 gm. dietary fiber, 75 RE vitamin A,
2 mg. vitamin C, 0 vitamin E as alpha tocopherol

Food exchange
1 vegetable, 4 lean meat, 1 1/2 bread/starch

Preparation time
20 minutes

Grilling time
15 minutes

DESSERTS

BAKED MACAROON PEACHES

4 servings, 2 peach halves each

4 peaches
2 Tbsp. sugar
4 coconut macaroon cookies, crushed
1 egg yolk or 1/4 cup liquid egg substitute
2 tsp. rum extract

Preheat oven to 350° F. Cut fresh peaches in half. Scoop
out 1 teaspoon of center pulp from each half. In a mixing
bowl, mash the pulp with sugar, macaroon crumbs, and egg
yolk. In a glass pie pan, place the peach halves close
together, cut side up. Spoon the macaroon mixture into
the center of each peach. Dot with rum extract. Bake for
20 minutes or until peaches are tender. Serve warm.

171 calories, 4 gm. fat (3 gm. fat with egg substitute), 2 gm. protein,
33 gm. carbohydrate, 53 mg. cholesterol with egg (0 with egg substitute), 60 mg. sodium, 2 gm. dietary fiber, 71 RE vitamin A,
5 mg. vitamin C, 0 vitamin E as alpha tocopherol

Food exchange
2 fruit, 1 fat

Preparation time
15 minutes

Baking time
20 minutes

BAVARIAN APRICOT MOLD

8 servings, 3/4 cup each

20-oz. can apricots
2 3-oz. pkg. pear or apricot flavored gelatin
2 cups boiling water
1 tsp. almond extract
1 cup nonfat peach yogurt
Garnish: toasted almonds

Drain apricots, reserving 2/3 cup juice. Chop apricots into small pieces and set aside. In a mixing bowl, dissolve gelatin in boiling water and then stir in reserved juice. Chill for 1 hour, until mixture is lightly thickened. Stir in almond extract, yogurt, and chopped apricots and pour into a 6-cup mold sprayed with nonstick cooking spray. Chill for at least 3 more hours or overnight. Loosen the gelatin dessert from the mold by dipping quickly in a shallow pan of hot water. Unmold onto a serving plate, and garnish with toasted almonds.

54 calories, 0 fat, 2 gm. protein, 11 gm. carbohydrate, 0 cholesterol, 25 mg. sodium, 0 dietary fiber, 130 RE vitamin A, 3 mg. vitamin C, 0.5 mg. vitamin E as alpha tocopherol

Food exchange
1 fruit

Preparation time
15 minutes

Chilling time
4 hours

BLUEBERRIES WITH PECAN SAUCE

4 servings, 3/4 cup each

3 cups fresh blueberries, washed and stems
   removed
1/2 cup nonfat sour cream
2 Tbsp. powdered sugar
2 Tbsp. orange juice
1 Tbsp. chopped pecans

Spoon berries into 4 fruit bowls. In a small container, combine sour cream, powdered sugar, orange juice, and pecans.
Pour over blueberries and serve.

127 calories, 2 gm. fat, 3 gm. protein, 24 gm. carbohydrate,
0 cholesterol, 39 mg. sodium, 0 dietary fiber, 45 RE vitamin A,
17 mg. vitamin C, 0 vitamin E as alpha tocopherol

Food exchange
1 fruit, 1/2 fat, 1/2 bread/starch

Preparation time
15 minutes

CARAMEL PEARS

8 servings, 1 pear each

2 Tbsp. margarine
1/2 cup sugar
8 medium pears, peeled, halved, and cored
Nonstick cooking spray
Garnish: nonfat frozen yogurt

Preheat oven to 450° F. Melt margarine in a 9- by 13-inch metal cake pan. Sprinkle 1/4 cup sugar in the pan. Place pear halves in the pan, cut side down. Sprinkle remaining sugar on top. Spray the pears with nonstick cooking spray. Bake for 20 minutes. Serve warm with nonfat frozen yogurt topping.

173 calories, 3 gm. fat, 0 protein, 37 gm. carbohydrate, 0 cholesterol, 36 mg. sodium, 4.4 gm. dietary fiber, 40 RE vitamin A, 6 mg. vitamin C, 0.8 mg. vitamin E as alpha tocopherol

Food exchange
2 fruit, 1 fat

Preparation time
15 minutes

Baking time
20 minutes

COUNTRY APPLE DELIGHT

8 servings, 1/8 of 8-inch baking dish

4 large eggs, beaten, or 1 cup liquid egg substitute
1 cup brown sugar
2/3 cup flour
1/4 cup wheat germ
2 tsp. baking powder
1/2 tsp. salt
3 Granny Smith apples, finely chopped
1 tsp. vanilla
2 Tbsp. chopped walnuts

Preheat oven to 375° F. In a large mixing bowl, combine eggs with brown sugar. Add flour, wheat germ, baking powder, and salt. Stir in apples and vanilla. Pour into an 8-inch square baking dish sprayed with nonstick cooking spray. Sprinkle the top with nuts. Bake for 45 minutes. Serve warm.

256 calories, 3 gm. fat with real egg (1 gm. with egg substitute),
5 gm. protein, 54 gm. carbohydrate, 88 mg. cholesterol with real egg
(0 cholesterol with egg substitute), 172 mg. sodium, 1.8 gm. dietary
fiber, 3 RE vitamin A, 3 mg. vitamin C, 0.6 mg. vitamin E as
alpha tocopherol

Food exchange
2 bread/starch, 1 1/2 fruit

Preparation time
20 minutes

Baking time
45 minutes

DREAMY AMARETTO FRUIT

4 servings, 1/2 cup each

2 Tbsp. Amaretto liqueur or 2 tsp. almond extract
2 Tbsp. dark brown sugar
1 cup nonfat sour cream
2 cups fresh fruit (strawberries and blueberries
  are best)
Cream

In a small mixing bowl, combine Amaretto and brown sugar until smooth. Add sour cream and mix well. Put fruit into 4 footed glass dishes. Drizzle with cream.

103 calories, 0 fat, 4 gm. protein, 21 gm. carbohydrate, 1 mg. cholesterol, 71 mg. sodium, 1.1 dietary fiber, 70 RE vitamin A, 26 mg. vitamin C, 0 vitamin E as alpha tocopherol

Food exchange
1/2 skim milk, 1 fruit

Preparation time
10 minutes

FRESH RASPBERRIES WITH GRAND MARNIER SAUCE

8 servings, 3/4 cup each

12 oz. evaporated skim milk
1 tsp. vanilla
2 large eggs or 1/2 cup liquid egg substitute
1/4 cup sugar
1/8 cup Grand Marnier liqueur or 2 tsp. orange
  extract
1 qt. fresh raspberries

In a heavy-bottomed saucepan over medium heat, scald evaporated skim milk and vanilla. Reduce heat to medium-low. In a small bowl, beat eggs with sugar until light yellow in color. Add egg mixture to the milk very slowly, stirring constantly over low heat until sauce thickens. Stir in liqueur or orange extract. Keep sauce in a container in the refrigerator up to 1 week. Serve 1/4 cup sauce over 1/2 cup raspberries.

106 calories, 1 gm. fat (0 fat with egg substitute), 5 gm. protein, 18 gm. carbohydrate, 44 mg. cholesterol with real egg (0 with egg substitute), 65 mg. sodium, 2.5 gm. dietary fiber, 81 RE vitamin A, 31 mg. vitamin C, 0 vitamin E as alpha tocopherol

Food exchange
1/2 skim milk, 1 fruit

Preparation time
20 minutes

FROZEN APRICOT CUPS

12 servings, 1 muffin cup each

2 8-oz. cartons nonfat orange or pineapple yogurt
17-oz. can apricot halves in juice, drained and
    cut up
1/4 cup chopped pecans

In a mixing bowl, stir together yogurt and apricots. Spoon
into paper-lined muffin cups. Sprinkle with pecans.
Cover and freeze until firm—at least 2 hours. Peel off
paper and serve in a fruit dish. These keep in the freezer
for up to a month.

74 calories, 3 gm. fat, 2 gm. protein, 9 gm. carbohydrate,
0 cholesterol, 30 mg. sodium, 0.4 gm. dietary fiber, 74 RE
vitamin A, 2 mg. vitamin C, 0.3 mg. vitamin E as alpha tocopherol

Food exchange
1/2 fat, 1 fruit

Preparation time
15 minutes

Freezing time:
at least 2 hours

FRENCH POACHED PEARS

8 servings, 1 whole pear each

8 ripe pears
2 cups cranberry-raspberry juice
1/2 cup water
1 cinnamon stick
Garnish: lemon wedges and small shortbread
cookies

Wash and peel the pears, leaving stems on whole pears. In
a heavy saucepan, combine all ingredients. Bring to a boil
uncovered. Reduce the heat, cover, and simmer for 15
minutes. Carefully lift pears into a serving bowl. Pour juice
over them. Refrigerate until well-chilled, at least 1 hour.
Spoon the juice over the pears twice during chilling. Serve
whole pears in fruit bowls, each garnished with a fresh
lemon wedge and a cookie.

129 calories, 0 fat, 0 protein, 33 gm. carbohydrate, 0 cholesterol,
2 mg. sodium, 1.8 gm. dietary fiber, 3 RE vitamin A,
24 mg. vitamin C, 0.8 mg. vitamin E as alpha tocopherol

Food exchange
2 fruit

Preparation time
10 minutes

Cooking time
20 minutes

Chilling time
1 hour

LIME PINEAPPLE FREEZE

12 servings, 1 muffin cup each

29-oz. can crushed pineapple in juice
3-oz. pkg. lime-flavored gelatin
1 cup marshmallows
1/2 tsp. peppermint flavoring
1 cup nonfat vanilla yogurt
Garnish: fresh mint

Drain pineapple well, reserving juice in a small saucepan. Bring pineapple juice to a boil and pour over lime gelatin in a large mixing bowl. Stir to fully dissolve gelatin; then add reserved pineapple, marshmallow, and peppermint flavoring. Cover and refrigerate for 30 minutes or until marshmallows soften. Fold in yogurt. Spoon mixture into paper-lined muffin cups. Cover and freeze until firm. Peel off paper and serve in a fruit dish. Garnish with fresh mint. These keep for 1 month in the freezer.

116 calories, 0 fat, 1 gm. protein, 28 gm. carbohydrate,
0 cholesterol, 23 mg. sodium, 0 dietary fiber, 2 RE vitamin A,
7 mg. vitamin C, 0 vitamin E as alpha tocopherol

Food exchange
2 fruit

Preparation time
15 minutes

Chilling time
30 minutes

Freezing time
at least 2 hours

MINTY MELON MARINADE

8 servings, 1/2 cup each

1 cantaloupe
1 honeydew melon
1/4 cup white creme de menthe
1/2 cup white wine cooler
1 tsp. poppy seeds
Garnish: reduced-fat vanilla sandwich cookie

Remove rinds from melons, scoop out seeds, and form balls from the flesh. Combine creme de menthe, wine cooler, and poppy seeds in a large salad bowl. Add melon balls to the mint marinade; cover and refrigerate at least 30 minutes or up to 24 hours before serving. Use a slotted spoon to serve the melon in fruit bowls. Garnish each serving with a sandwich cookie.

83 calories, 0 fat, 1 gm. protein, 20 gm. carbohydrate, 0 cholesterol, 22 mg. sodium, 0 dietary fiber, 221 RE vitamin A, 68 mg. vitamin C, 0 vitamin E as alpha tocopherol

Food exchange
1 1/2 fruit

Preparation time
15 minutes

Chilling time
30 minutes to 24 hours

NECTARINES FOR COMPANY

8 servings, 3/4 cup each

1 cup skim milk
2 tsp. finely grated orange peel
1/4 cup sugar
1 1/2 Tbsp. cornstarch
2 beaten eggs or 1/2 cup liquid egg substitute
1 tsp. orange extract
6 ripe, but firm nectarines, sliced into 8 sections
Garnish: fresh raspberries or red grapes

Combine milk and orange peel in a small saucepan and bring just to a simmer. Remove from heat and set aside. In a small bowl, mix sugar with cornstarch and beaten eggs. Slowly whisk hot milk into the egg mixture. Return the mixture to the saucepan and cook until thickened, about 5 minutes. Remove from heat and add orange extract. Transfer to a metal bowl to speed chilling, and refrigerate for at least 1 hour. To serve, spoon the chilled sauce on a dessert plate. Top with sliced nectarines, fanning them around the plate. Garnish with a fresh raspberry or a small cluster of red grapes.

100 calories, 1 gm. fat with egg (0 with egg substitute), 5 gm. protein, 22 gm. carbohydrate, 4 mg. cholesterol with real egg (0 with egg substitute), 29 mg. sodium, 1.4 gm. dietary fiber, 93 RE vitamin A, 11 mg. vitamin C, 0 vitamin E as alpha tocopherol

Food exchange
1 1/2 fruit

Preparation time
20 minutes

Chilling time
1 hour

PEACH SHERBET DESSERT

8 servings, 1/8 of 8-inch square pan each

3-oz. pkg. nonfat cream cheese, softened
1/4 cup reduced-fat mayonnaise
2 cups orange or lemon sherbet
11-oz. can mandarin orange sections, drained and
  cut up
16-oz. can peach slices, drained and chopped
Garnish: dried pineapple chunks

In a large mixing bowl, beat together softened cream
cheese and mayonnaise. Stir sherbet to soften, and fold
into cream cheese mixture. Stir in fruit, and transfer to an
8-inch square pan. Cover and freeze until firm, about 2
hours. Cut and serve. Garnish squares of dessert with dried
pineapple chunks. This dessert will keep in the freezer for
up to 1 month.

144 calories, 1 gm. fat, 2 gm. protein, 33 gm. carbohydrate, 3 mg.
cholesterol, 131 mg. sodium, 1.2 gm. dietary fiber, 51 RE vitamin A,
22 mg. vitamin C, 0 vitamin E as alpha tocopherol

Food exchange
1 bread/starch, 1 fruit

Preparation time
20 minutes

Freezing time
at least 2 hours

PEAR LIME TOWER

8 servings, 3/4 cup each

2 3-oz. pkg. sugar-free lime gelatin
1 cup boiling water
1 6-oz. can frozen lemonade concentrate
6 large ice cubes
4 small pears, halved and cored
8 whole strawberries
Garnish: 1/2 cup nonfat sour cream
1/2 tsp. finely grated lemon peel

Combine gelatin with boiling water in a mixing bowl. Stir to fully dissolve gelatin. Add frozen lemonade concentrate and ice cubes and stir again. Select 8 large fluted wine goblets or tumblers to form the gelatin towers. Pour about 1/4 cup of the gelatin mixture into the goblets and refrigerate for 1 hour, until partially set. Place a whole strawberry into the middle of the pear half and press a pear half down into the partially set gelatin. Pour remaining gelatin over the pears. Chill again for at least 2 hours. Unmold the towers by running each goblet under hot water for a few seconds and turning out onto a salad plate. Garnish the top of the tower with 1 tablespoon of nonfat sour cream and a sprinkle of lemon peel.

115 calories, 0 fat, 1 gm. protein, 28 gm. carbohydrate,
0 cholesterol, 21 mg. sodium, 1.8 gm. dietary fiber, 20 RE vitamin A,
18 mg. vitamin C, 0.3 mg. vitamin E as alpha tocopherol

Food exchange
2 fruit

Preparation time
20 minutes

Chilling time
3 hours

PRETTY POLYNESIAN FRUIT PLATE

8 servings, 3/4 cup each

1 fresh pineapple
3 kiwifruit, peeled and sliced
1 mango, peeled and sliced
1 papaya, peeled and formed into balls
1/4 cup chopped pistachios
Optional dressing: pina colada yogurt

Cut the top off the pineapple, then cut in half lengthwise. Cut each half into 8 or 9 slices. Choose a pretty oval platter and layer fruits: pineapple slices on the bottom, then kiwi, mango slices, papaya balls, and finally, sprinkle with chopped pistachios. Serve as a pretty ending to a meal with an optional dressing of pina colada yogurt.

124 calories, 4 gm. fat, 2 gm. protein, 22 gm. carbohydrate, 0 cholesterol, 3 mg. sodium, 3.4 gm. dietary fiber, 165 RE vitamin A, 69 mg. vitamin C, 0.5 mg. vitamin E as alpha tocopherol

Food exchange
1 fat, 1 1/2 fruit

Preparation time
20 minutes

RASPBERRY CREME PIE

8 servings, 1/8 pie each

9-inch prepared graham cracker crust
1 quart fresh raspberries, washed, and drained
    (reserve 1/2 cup berries for garnish)
2/3 cup sugar
3 Tbsp. cornstarch
1 1/2 cups cranberry-raspberry juice
3-oz. pkg. sugar-free raspberry gelatin
8 oz. nonfat vanilla yogurt
1/4 cup nonfat cream cheese, softened

Place berries in prepared crust. In a medium saucepan, mix sugar and cornstarch. Gradually stir in cranberry-raspberry juice until smooth. Cook over medium heat, stirring constantly, until mixture comes to a boil. Boil for 1 minute, then stir in gelatin until fully dissolved. Cool to room temperature, then pour gelatin mixture over berries. Refrigerate. Mix yogurt with softened cream cheese and spread over the pie before serving. Garnish the top of the pie with reserved berries.

206 calories, 1 gm. fat, 3 gm. protein, 45 gm. carbohydrate,
0 cholesterol, 94 mg. sodium, 1.6 gm. dietary fiber, 16 RE vitamin A,
29 mg. vitamin C, 0 vitamin E as alpha tocopherol

Food exchange
2 fruit, 1 bread/starch

Preparation time
20 minutes

Chilling time
2 hours

RHUBARB CUSTARD PIE

8 servings, 1/8 pie each

1 prepared graham cracker crust
2/3 cup sugar
1 tsp. margarine
1 large egg or 1/4 cup liquid egg substitute
2 egg whites
1/4 cup skim milk
1 tsp. almond extract
6 cups chopped rhubarb
2 Tbsp. flour
1/4 cup all fruit strawberry preserves

In a mixing bowl, beat together sugar, margarine, egg, egg whites, milk, and almond extract until smooth. In another bowl, mix rhubarb with flour. Fold rhubarb into the egg mixture, and turn into the prepared pie crust. Bake for 1 hour, until the filling is firm. Top with strawberry preserves.

171 calories, 1 gm. fat (0 with egg substitute), 3 gm. protein, 35 gm. carbohydrate, 22 mg. cholesterol with egg (0 with egg substitute), 109 mg. sodium, 1.4 gm. dietary fiber, 31 RE vitamin A, 7 mg. vitamin C, 0 vitamin E as alpha tocopherol

Food exchange
1 1/2 fruit, 1 bread/starch

Preparation time
15 minutes

Baking time
1 hour

STRAWBERRY-BANANA DELIGHT

12 servings, 1/12 cake with 1/2 cup fruit and
1/4 cup ice milk

3 cups reduced-fat baking mix (Bisquick Light®)
1 cup plus 2 Tbsp. buttermilk
2 Tbsp. vegetable oil
1 Tbsp. vanilla
1 qt. fresh strawberries, washed, hulled, and sliced
4 bananas, peeled and sliced
1 Tbsp. lemon juice
2 Tbsp. sugar
3 cups ice milk

Preheat oven to 425° F. Spray an 11- by 7-inch baking pan
with nonstick cooking spray. In a mixing bowl, combine
baking mix, buttermilk, oil, and vanilla just until blended.
Spoon batter into the prepared pan and bake for 15 minutes. Cool shortcake for 10 minutes, then remove from the
pan. Meanwhile, combine berries with sliced bananas,
lemon juice, and sugar. Spoon fruit over slices of cake, and
top each serving with 1/4 cup ice milk.

189 calories, 3 gm. fat, 5 gm. protein, 38 gm. carbohydrate,
8 mg. cholesterol, 74 mg. sodium, 1.6 gm. dietary fiber, 32 RE vitamin A, 32 mg. vitamin C, 0.5 mg. vitamin E as alpha tocopherol

Food exchange
1 bread/starch, 1 fat, 1 fruit

Preparation time
15 minutes

Baking time
15 minutes

Cooling time
10 minutes

SPICY ORANGES AND DATES

8 servings, 1/2 cup each

1/2 cup orange juice
2 cinnamon sticks
10 whole cloves
3 large oranges, peeled, sectioned, and snipped
    into small pieces
1 cup chopped dates

In a small saucepan, combine orange juice with cinnamon
and cloves. Bring to a boil. Meanwhile, combine orange
pieces and chopped dates in a salad bowl. Pour hot liquid
over the fruit and cover. Chill for at least 30 minutes. Use
this as a topping for reduced-fat yellow cake or lemon cus-
tard angel food cake.

110 calories, 0 fat, 1 gm. protein, 28 gm. carbohydrate, 0 cholesterol, 1 mg. sodium, 2.2 gm. dietary fiber, 15 RE vitamin A,
30 mg. vitamin C, 0 vitamin E as alpha tocopherol

Food exchange
2 fruit

Preparation time
15 minutes

Chilling time
30 minutes

STRAWBERRY SOUFFLE

8 servings, 3/4 cup each

1 quart fresh strawberries
2 3-oz. pkg. strawberry-flavored gelatin
1 cup boiling water
1 cup sugar-free lemon-lime soft drink
3 oz. nonfat cream cheese, softened
1/4 cup reduced-fat mayonnaise
Garnish: 1/4 cup chopped pecans

Wash strawberries and use a food chopper to chop fine. In a mixing bowl, combine gelatin with boiling water, stirring to completely dissolve gelatin. Add soft drink, and stir again. Add softened cream cheese and mayonnaise and use a whisk to stir smooth. Refrigerate for 30 minutes. After chilling, fold in chopped berries. Turn mixture into a souffle dish and garnish with pecans. Refrigerate until firm (about 2 hours). Loosen the souffle by gently dipping the dish in a shallow pan of warm water. Slice and serve on dessert plates.

85 calories, 5 gm. fat, 1 gm. protein, 9 gm. carbohydrate, 0 cholesterol, 104 mg. sodium, 1 gm. dietary fiber, 16 RE vitamin A, 42 mg. vitamin C, 3.3 mg. vitamin E as alpha tocopherol (with chopped almonds)

Food exchange
1 fat, 1/2 fruit

Preparation time
20 minutes

Chilling time
2 hours, 30 minutes

JUST FOR KIDS

AFTER-SCHOOL BAKED APPLES

4 servings, 1/2 cup each

2 large baking apples (Rome, Jonathan, or
MacIntosh are best)
2 Tbsp. water
2 Tbsp. brown sugar
1/4 cup grape jelly or strawberry jam

Core and cut apples into very thin slices. Place apple slices
in an 8-inch square microwave-safe baking dish. Sprinkle
with water and brown sugar. Dot grape jelly or strawberry
jam over the apples. Cover with plastic wrap and
microwave on high power for 7 to 9 minutes. Check apples
for doneness with a fork. They should be tender, not
tough. Cool and serve.

115 calories, 0 fat, 0 protein, 28 gm. carbohydrate, 0 cholesterol,
3 mg. sodium, 2.8 gm. dietary fiber, 3 RE vitamin A, 3 mg. vitamin
C, 0.6 mg. vitamin E as alpha tocopherol

Food exchange
2 fruit

Preparation time
10 minutes

Baking time
10 minutes

BANANA PIE

8 servings, 1/8 pie each

9-inch prepared graham cracker crust
3-oz. pkg. sugar-free chocolate pudding
2 cups skim milk, divided
4 large bananas
3-oz. pkg. sugar-free vanilla pudding
Garnish: chocolate curls

In a medium saucepan, combine 1 cup skim milk with chocolate pudding mix. Cook over medium-high heat until thick. Pour pudding into prepared crust. Wash the saucepan out, and repeat the procedure with the vanilla pudding and remaining 1 cup of skim milk. Slice bananas and place on top of chocolate pudding layer. Pour vanilla pudding over the top of the bananas and refrigerate for 2 hours. Garnish the pie with curls of hard chocolate.

151 calories, 3 gm. fat, 2 gm. protein, 29 gm. carbohydrate,
2 mg. cholesterol, 197 mg. sodium, 1.6 gm. dietary fiber,
36 RE vitamin A, 5 mg. vitamin C, 0 vitamin E as alpha tocopherol

Food exchange
1 fat, 1/2 fruit, 1 bread/starch

Preparation time
15 minutes

Chilling time
2 hours

BANANAS ON A STICK

4 servings, 1 banana each

4 large firm bananas
8 flat wooden sticks
3-oz. pkg. instant chocolate pudding
1 cup skim milk
1/2 cup Grape Nuts® cereal

Mix skim milk with pudding mix in a covered jar or shaker container for 2 minutes, until thick. Peel bananas and slice 1/2 inch off the pointed end of each. Insert a flat wooden stick into the trimmed end. Pour pudding out into a shallow pie pan and pour Grape Nuts into another shallow pie pan. Roll the bananas into the pudding and then into the Grape Nuts. Pass out to the troops and enjoy!

237 calories, 0 fat, 7 gm. protein, 54 gm. carbohydrate, 0 cholesterol, 240 mg. sodium, 2.4 gm. dietary fiber, 420 RE vitamin A, 11 mg. vitamin C, 0 vitamin E as alpha tocopherol

Food exchange
2 1/2 fruit, 1 skim milk

Preparation time
15 minutes

BANANA SOUP

8 servings, 6 oz. each

6 bananas
2 Tbsp. lemon juice
1 tsp. cinnamon
1/2 tsp. nutmeg
1/4 tsp. ground cloves
1 cup skim milk
1/4 cup raisins

Blend the first 6 ingredients in a blender on high speed for 3 minutes. Chill in a metal bowl for 1 hour. Pour into soup bowls and top with raisins. To reduce chilling time, plan ahead and put your bananas in the refrigerator until ready to prepare.

105 calories, 0 fat, 2 gm. protein, 25 gm. carbohydrate, 0 cholesterol, 17 mg. sodium, 2.6 gm. dietary fiber, 25 RE vitamin A, 9 mg. vitamin C, 0 vitamin E as alpha tocopherol

Food exchange
2 fruit

Preparation time
15 minutes

BIRTHDAY PARTY FANTASY SUNDAES

Let everyone create their own fantasy, or choose from the six below.

8 servings, 1 cup ice milk and 1/2 cup of fruit

TRADITIONAL:

> 2 qt. vanilla ice milk
> 4 large bananas, peeled and sliced
> 1 cup sliced strawberries
> 1/2 cup chocolate syrup

413 calories, 9 gm. fat, 9 gm. protein, 75 gm. carbohydrate, 30 mg. cholesterol, 200 mg. sodium, 2 gm. dietary fiber, 111 RE vitamin A, 17 mg. vitamin C, 0 vitamin E as alpha tocopherol

Food exchange
2 1/2 bread/starch, 3 fruit, 1 fat

HAWAIIAN:

> 2 qt. rainbow sherbet
> 1 cup crushed pineapple, well drained
> 1/4 cup coconut

354 calories, 3 gm. fat, 2 gm. protein, 78 gm. carbohydrate, 13 mg. cholesterol, 84 mg. sodium, 0 dietary fiber, 0 vitamin A, 2 mg. vitamin C, 0 vitamin E as alpha tocopherol

Food exchange
3 fruit, 2 bread/starch

ELEGANT RASPBERRY:

2 qt. chocolate frozen yogurt
2 cup fresh raspberries
1/2 cup chocolate syrup

400 calories, 0 fat, 10 gm. protein, 87 gm. carbohydrate, 0 cholesterol, 180 mg. sodium, 0 dietary fiber, 4 RE vitamin A,
7 mg. vitamin C, 0 vitamin E as alpha tocopherol

Food exchange
2 bread/starch, 1 1/2 skim milk, 2 fruit

CARAMEL APPLE:

2 qt. butter brickle ice milk
1/2 cup raisins
1/2 cup hot applesauce
1/2 cup caramel topping

416 calories, 9 gm. fat, 1 gm. protein, 82 gm. carbohydrate, 32 mg.
cholesterol, 192 mg. sodium, 0 dietary fiber, 0 vitamin A,
0 vitamin C, 0 vitamin E as alpha tocopherol

Food exchange
2 bread/starch, 1 skim milk, 1 fat, 1 1/2 fruit

VERY BERRY:

2 qt. strawberry frozen yogurt
1 cup blueberries
1 cup strawberries, halved
1/2 cup all fruit raspberry preserves, warmed

354 calories, 5 gm. fat, 11 gm. protein, 67 gm. carbohydrate, 14 mg.
cholesterol, 335 mg. sodium, 0 dietary fiber, 2 RE vitamin A, 12
mg. vitamin C, 0 vitamin E as alpha tocopherol

Food exchange
1 skim milk, 1 fat, 2 bread/starch, 1 fruit

NUTTY ALL THE WAY:

2 qt. maple nut ice milk
1/4 cup dried apricots, diced
1/4 cup dried pineapple, diced
1/4 cup Grape Nuts® cereal

368 calories, 10 gm. fat, 10 gm. protein, 61 gm. carbohydrate, 34
mg. cholesterol, 162 mg. sodium, 0 dietary fiber, 76 RE vitamin A,
0 vitamin C, 0 vitamin E as alpha tocopherol

Food exchange
1 fat, 1 skim milk, 2 bread/starch, 1 fruit

Preparation time
10 minutes

BROILED SUNSHINE

4 servings, 1/2 grapefruit each

2 large red grapefruit
2 Tbsp. maple syrup

Cut the grapefruit in half and remove the seeds. Cut between each section for easy removal. Place halves on a metal baking sheet and place under the broiler for 6 to 8 minutes, until the top of the fruit starts to brown. Drizzle the top of the fruit with maple syrup. Serve.

63 calories, 0 fat, 0 protein, 16 gm. carbohydrate, 0 cholesterol, 1 mg. sodium, 2.4 gm. dietary fiber, 32 RE vitamin A, 46 mg. vitamin C, 0 vitamin E as alpha tocopherol

Food exchange
1 fruit

Preparation time
10 minutes

Broiling time
6 to 8 minutes

CHEESY GREEN BEANS

4 servings, 1/2 cup each

16-oz. can green beans, drained
1/2 cup soft cheese spread (such as Cheez Whiz®)

Drain beans and pour into a small microwave-safe bowl.
Add soft cheese and microcook on high power for 2 minutes. Stir to mix. Tastes good at lunchtime with peanut
butter sandwiches.

101 calories, 6 gm. fat, 5 gm. protein, 7 gm. carbohydrate,
20 mg. cholesterol, 753 mg. sodium (to reduce sodium, use no-
added-salt green beans), 2 gm. dietary fiber, 99 RE vitamin A,
5 mg. vitamin C, 0 vitamin E as alpha tocopherol

Food exchange
2 vegetable, 1 fat

Preparation time
10 minutes

E L I Z A B E T H ' S   P O P S I C L E S ®

8 servings, 1 stick each

12-oz. can frozen cranberry-raspberry juice
concentrate
2 cups water

Combine juice concentrate with water. Pour into 8 plastic
Popsicle® molds. Freeze until firm.

66 calories, 0 fat, 0 protein, 16 gm. carbohydrate, 0 cholesterol,
2 mg. sodium, 0 dietary fiber, 0 vitamin A, 31 mg. vitamin C,
0 vitamin E as alpha tocopherol

Food exchange
1 fruit

Preparation time
15 minutes

Freezing time
2 hours

FROZEN GRAPES ON THE GO

Teenagers hungry 15 minutes before dinner? Give them a handful of frozen grapes. (Whole grapes are not recommended for small children.)

4 servings, 1/2 cup each

1 large bunch green grapes

Wash grapes and remove from the stem. Trim any brown ends. Place grapes on a flat baking sheet and freeze for 30 minutes. Transfer to a jar for long-term freezer storage.

75 calories, 0 fat, 0 protein, 20 gm. carbohydrate, 0 cholesterol, 0 sodium, 0.6 gm. dietary fiber, 10 RE vitamin A, 5 mg. vitamin C, 0 vitamin E as alpha tocopherol

Food exchange
1 fruit

Preparation time
15 minutes

Freezing time
30 minutes

FRUIT-JUICE JIGGLERS®

8 servings, 1/4 cup each

2 cups apricot nectar
3 3-oz. pkg. sugar-free raspberry gelatin

In a small saucepan, bring nectar to a boil. Meanwhile,
pour gelatin into a small mixing bowl. Pour boiling nectar
over gelatin, and stir to dissolve. Pour mixture into an 8-
inch square pan, chill for 2 hours or until firm, and cut
into 8 small squares.

35 calories, 0 fat, 0 protein, 9 gm. carbohydrate, 0 cholesterol,
1 mg. sodium, 0 dietary fiber, 1187 RE vitamin A, 4 mg. vitamin C,
0 vitamin E as alpha tocopherol

Food exchange
1/2 fruit

Preparation time
15 minutes

Chilling time
2 hours

GOOD FOR YOU LEMONADE

8 servings, 1 cup each

2 qt. orange juice
2 1-qt. pkg. sugar-free Koolaid® lemonade mix

Combine ingredients in a 2-quart pitcher and serve at snack time.

101 calories, 0 fat, 1 gm. protein, 24 gm. carbohydrate,
0 cholesterol, 14 mg. sodium, 0 dietary fiber, 14 RE vitamin A,
74 mg. vitamin C, 0 vitamin E as alpha tocopherol

Food exchange
2 fruit

Preparation time
5 minutes

JONATHAN'S APPLES

Jonathan Wick showed us this trick!

4 servings, 1/2 apple each

1/4 cup sugar
1 tsp. cinnamon
2 large Red Delicious apples, sliced into wedges

Combine cinnamon and sugar in a small bowl. Pour out onto 4 salad plates. Divide apple wedges among the 4 plates. Let kids dip the apple slices into the cinnamon-sugar mixture.

129 calories, 0 fat, 0 protein, 33 gm. carbohydrate, 0 cholesterol, 1 mg. sodium, 2.8 gm. dietary fiber, 7 RE vitamin A, 7 mg. vitamin C, 0.6 mg. vitamin E as alpha tocopherol

Food exchange
2 fruit

Preparation time
15 minutes

MINI VEGETABLE PIZZAS

Use your favorite fresh veggies to top these pizzas!

8 servings, 2 muffin halves each

8 English muffins, split
Nonstick cooking spray
8 oz. reduced-fat spaghetti sauce (such as Today's
  Recipe by Ragu®)
4 scallions, sliced thin
1 green pepper, chopped fine
8 mushrooms, sliced thin
4 oz. part-skim mozzarella cheese, shredded

Preheat broiler. Place muffin halves on a baking sheet.
Spray generously with non-stick cooking spray. Place under
the broiler for 5 minutes. Remove and top with sauce, scallions, chopped pepper, sliced mushrooms, and shredded
cheese. Return to the broiler for 7 to 10 more minutes,
until cheese is well melted.

216 calories, 4 gm. fat, 9 gm. protein, 34 gm. carbohydrate,
8 mg. cholesterol, 485 mg. sodium, 2 gm. dietary fiber, 86 RE vitamin A, 31 mg. vitamin C, 0 vitamin E as alpha tocopherol

Food exchange
1/2 lean meat, 2 bread/starch, 1 vegetable

Preparation time
10 minutes

Broiling time
15 minutes

PURPLE COW

4 servings, 1 cup each

2 cups purple grape juice
1 cup non-fat frozen vanilla yogurt

Combine ingredients in a blender container. Blend until smooth and pour out into 4 tumblers.

156 calories, 0 fat, 2 gm. protein, 37 gm. carbohydrate, 0 cholesterol, 38 mg. sodium, 0 dietary fiber, 1 RE vitamin A, 0 vitamin C, 0 vitamin E as alpha tocopherol

Food exchange
2 fruit, 1/2 skim milk

Preparation time
10 minutes

G·IFTS

DRIED FRUIT GIFT PACK

Friend in the hospital? Share this fruity treat instead of flowers or chocolate.

32 1-oz. servings

1 3-lb. coffee can with a lid
1 yd. pretty fabric
1/2 lb. dried apricots
1/2 lb. dried pears
1/2 lb. dried apples

Clean coffee can well. Lay the fabric out on a table, printed side down and place the can in the center. Wrap the fabric up around the can and press the edges down into the middle. Place a clear plastic bag in the can, on top of the fabric. Layer bits of dried fruit into the bag. Close the bag with a twist tie. Place cover on the can.

83 calories, 0 fat, 1 gm. protein, 21 gm. carbohydrate, 0 cholesterol, 3 mg. sodium, 3 gm. dietary fiber, 126 RE vitamin A, 1 mg. vitamin C, 0 vitamin E

Food exchange
1 1/2 fruit

Preparation time
20 minutes

LAZY WAY PICKLES

8 pints, 64 1/4-cup servings

4 cups sugar
1/2 cup salt
1 qt. vinegar
1 pt. water
24 slices white onion
4 qt. fresh pickling cucumbers
4 tsp. celery seed
4 tsp. dill seed
2 tsp. alum

Bring sugar, salt, vinegar, and water to a boil. Meanwhile, clean and stem cucumbers. Quarter the cucumbers and fit into 8 pint jars. Add 3 slices of onion to each jar. Add 1/2 tsp. dill seed, 1/2 tsp. celery seed, and 1/4 tsp. alum to each pint. Pour in boiling syrup, stopping 1/2 inch from the top of the jar; cover with lids. Refrigerate for 2 weeks. Then enjoy.

61 calories, 0 fat, 0 protein, 15 gm. carbohydrate, 0 cholesterol, 756 mg. sodium, 0 dietary fiber, 12 RE vitamin A, 3 mg. vitamin C, 0 vitamin E

Food exchange
1 fruit

Preparation time
30 minutes

Refrigeration time
2 weeks

MAKE YOUR OWN FRUIT BASKET

> 1 grape, strawberry, or peach crate or box (Ask
> the produce keeper at your favorite store.
> Crates are usually free for the asking.)
> Wrapping paper to suit the occasion: Valentines,
> Birthday, New Baby, etc.
> 2 large grapefruit
> 4 oranges
> 1 lb. Granny Smith apples
> 1 lb. Red Delicious apples
> 1 lb. pears
> 1 lb. red or green grapes, cut into 3 clusters
> 5 bananas, preferably in 1 cluster
> 1 kiwifruit
> *Garnish:* fresh strawberries, apricots, or
> bing cherries.

Cover the crate or box with wrapping paper. Layer fruit in
order given. Add a few fresh strawberries, apricots, or bing
cherries to the top. You may wish to cover the whole box
in colored plastic food wrap and attach a decorative bow
for extra-special delivery.

MARY FORD'S SALSA

8 pints, 32 1/2-cup servings

16 cups peeled and chopped tomatoes
4 cups chopped green peppers
4 1/2 cups chopped jalapeno peppers
4 cups chopped white or yellow onions
3 Tbsp. salt
12 cloves garlic, minced
3 cups cider vinegar
1/4 cup sugar

Combine vegetables with salt and minced garlic in a large stockpot. Simmer uncovered over medium-low heat for 3 hours, stirring occasionally. Add vinegar and sugar, stir to dissolve, and ladle into 8 sterile pint jars. Place sterile covers on jars, and refrigerate until ready to use or process 30 minutes in a boiling water bath for room-temperature storage. Use as a topping on grilled chicken breasts, as a sauce for scrambled eggs or for dipping with vegetables or reduced-fat chips.

Note: If you prefer chunky-style salsa, add onions and peppers during the last 30 minutes of simmering, before the vinegar and sugar.

58 calories, 0 fat, 1 gm. protein, 13 gm. carbohydrate, 0 cholesterol, 1077 mg. sodium (To decrease sodium, reduce salt to 1 tablespoon.), 1.4 gm. dietary fiber, 143 RE vitamin A, 52 mg. vitamin C, 0 vitamin E

Food exchange
2 vegetable

Preparation time
20 minutes

Cooking time
3 hours

MAY DAY SURPRISE

1 3-pack of Better Boy tomato plants
1 3-pack of California Wonder green bell peppers
1 small sack of onion sets
1 fresh flowering plant

Find a flat, shallow straw basket. Visit your favorite plant outlet and put together an invitation to garden.

PICKLED BEETS

These are lovely to behold. The color calls for Christmas giving.

8 pints or 64 1/4-cup servings

1 gallon beets
2 cups sugar
1 tsp. salt
1 Tbsp. whole allspice
3 1/2 cups vinegar
1 1/2 cups water
8 cinnamon sticks

Prepare beets by washing well and cutting off the top greens, leaving just 1 inch of stem. Cut off the roots. Place in a large kettle of boiling water, and simmer for 20 minutes or until tender. Drain well and remove the skins. Slice beets back into the kettle. Add sugar, spices, vinegar, and water. Heat through to dissolve sugar. Place a cinnamon stick in each pint jar; add beets and syrup and cover with lids. Refrigerate until ready to use, or process in a boiling water bath for 30 minutes to seal for room-temperature storage.

51 calories, 0 fat, 0 protein, 12 gm. carbohydrate, 0 cholesterol, 76 mg. sodium, 1.1 dietary fiber, 1 RE vitamin A, 1 mg. vitamin C, 0 vitamin E

Food exchange
1 fruit

Preparation time
30 minutes

Cooking time
20 minutes

REFRIGERATOR RELISH

8 pints of relish, 64 1/4-cup servings

2 medium heads of cabbage
4 carrots
4 red peppers
4 green peppers
12 onions
1/2 cup salt
6 cups vinegar
6 cups sugar
1 Tbsp. mustard seed
1 Tbsp. celery seed

In a food processor, chop cabbage, carrots, peppers, and onion to a relish consistency. Place in a large bowl or container; add salt to vegetables and stir well. Allow mixture to sit for 2 hours at room temperature, then drain well. Add remaining ingredients and pack into clean pint jars. Place covers on the jars and refrigerate. This relish is ready in 1 week.

107 calories, 0 fat, 1 gm. protein, 27 gm. carbohydrate,
0 cholesterol, 762 mg. sodium, 1.2 gm. dietary fiber,
142 RE vitamin A, 50 mg. vitamin C, 0 vitamin E

Food exchange
1 1/2 fruit, 1 vegetable

Preparation time
30 minutes

Marinating time
2 hours

Refrigeration time
1 week

SELMA'S DILLY BEANS

4 quarts, 64 1/4-cup servings

4 qt. fresh green beans (may even use the thick
   woody variety that come at the end of the garden season)
2 gallons water
10 cloves fresh garlic
15 whole peppercorns
15 heads fresh dill
5 cups water
1/2 cup pickling salt
1/2 cup vinegar

Wash beans well and remove stems. Boil 2 gallons of water
in a large kettle. Add beans to boiling water and simmer
for 10 minutes. Drain. Pack into sterilized quart jars. Add 3
heads of fresh dill, 3 peppercorns and 2 cloves of garlic to
each quart. In the same kettle, bring the 5 cups of water,
pickling salt, and vinegar to a boil. Pour over beans. Seal
with tight-fitting lids and store in the refrigerator for 3
weeks; then they are ready to eat. Decorate with yellow
ribbons for gifts.

8 calories, 0 fat, 0 protein, 2 gm. carbohydrate, 0 cholesterol,
756 mg. sodium, 0 dietary fiber, 18 RE vvitamin C,
0 vitamin E as alpha tocopherol

Food exchange
Free

Preparation time
30 minutes

SCHOOL DAYS PACKAGE FROM GRANDMA

Think of your grandchildren in August with an assortment of good-for-you brown bag goodies.

Small boxes of raisins
Yogurt-covered raisins
Juice boxes
Dried apricots
Dried apples
Fruit leather
Dried pineapple
Dried pears
Banana chips
Individual cans of Mexican-flavored vegetable
   juice cocktail

THANKSGIVING HOSTESS GIFT

1 large straw cornucopia
1 small acorn squash
3 fresh sweet potatoes or yams
4 miniature green and yellow gourds
1/2 lb. assorted nuts in the shells

Arrange the vegetables in the cornucopia. Garnish with nuts. Take along for your Thanksgiving hostess.

INDEX

Other Best-Selling Cookbooks by Author M.J. Smith

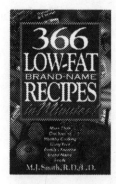

366 Low-Fat Brand-Name Recipes in Minutes

by M.J. Smith, M.S., R.D./L.D.

Here's more than a year's worth of the fastest family favorites using the country's most popular brand-name foods—from Minute Rice® to Ore Ida®—while reducing unwanted calories, fat, salt, and cholesterol.

004247   ISBN 1-56561-050-4 $12.95   ❏

All-American Low-Fat Meals in Minutes

by M.J. Smith R.D., L.D., M.A.

Filled with tantalizing recipes and valuable tips, this cookbook makes great-tasting low-fat foods a snap for holidays, special occasions, or everyday. Most recipes take only minutes to prepare.

004079   ISBN 0-937721-73-5 $12.95   ❏

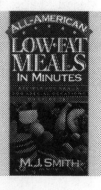

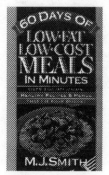

60 Days of Low-Fat, Low-Cost Meals in Minutes

by M.J. Smith, R.D., L.D., M.A.

Following the path of the best-seller *All American Low-Fat Meals in Minutes*, here are more than 150 quick and sumptuous recipes complete with the latest exchange values and nutrition facts for lowering calories, fat, salt, and cholesterol. This book contains complete menus for 60 days and recipes that use ingredients found in virtually any grocery store—most for a total cost of less than $10.

004205   ISBN 1-56561-010-5 $12.95   ❏

CHRONIMED PUBLISHING
BOOKS OF RELATED INTEREST

Fight Fat & Win Cookbook by Elaine Moquette-Magee, M.P.H., R.D. Now you can give up fat and create great tasting foods without giving up your busy lifestyle. Born from the bestseller *Fight Fat & Win*, this practical cookbook shows you how to make more than 150 easy and tempting snacks, breakfasts, lunches, dinners, and desserts that your family will never know contain little or no fat.

004254   ISBN 1-56561-055-5 $12.95   ❏

Fight Fat and Win, Updated & Revised Edition by Elaine Moquette-Magee, R.D., M.P.H. This breakthrough book explains how to easily incorporate low-fat dietary guidelines into every modern eating experience, from fast food and common restaurants to quick meals at home, simply by making smarter choices.

004244   ISBN 1-56561-047-4 $9.95   ❏

Fast Food Facts, Revised and Expanded Edition by Marion Franz, R.D., M.S. This revised and up-to-date best-seller shows how to make smart nutrition choices at fast food restaurants—and tells what to avoid. Includes complete nutrition information of more than 1,500 menu offerings from the 37 largest fast food chains.

Standard-size edition, 004240   ISBN 1-56561-043-1 $7.95   ❏
Pocket edition, 004228   ISBN 1-56561-031-8 $4.95   ❏

Convenience Food Facts by Arlene Monk, R.D., C.D.E., with an introduction by Marion Franz, R.D., M.S. Includes complete nutrition information, tips, and exchange values on more than 1,500 popular name brand processed foods commonly found in grocery store freezers and shelves. Helps you plan easy-to-prepare, nutritious meals.

004081   ISBN 0-937721-77-8 $10.95   ❏

The Brand-Name Guide to Low-Fat and Fat-Free Foods by J. Michael Lapchick with Rosa Mo, R.D., Ed.D. For the first time in one easy-to-swallow guide is a compendium of just about every brand-name food available containing little or no fat—with complete nutrition information.

004242   ISBN 1-56561-045-8 $9.95   ❑

Muscle Pain Relief in 90 Seconds by Dale Anderson, M.D. Now you're only 90 seconds away from relieving your muscle pain—drug free! From back pain and shin splints to headaches and tennis elbow, Dr. Anderson's innovative "Fold and Hold" technique can help. Simple, safe, and painless, this method is a must for all of us with muscle aches and twinges.

004257   ISBN 1-56561-058-X $10.95 ❑

Taking the Work Out of Working Out by Charles Roy Schroeder, Ph.D. This breakthrough guide shows how to easily convert what many consider to be a chore into enjoyable, creative, and sensual experiences that you'll look forward to. Includes methods for every form of exercise—including aerobics, weight lifting, jogging, dance, and more!
•A Doubleday Health Book Club Selection

004246   ISBN 1-56561-049-0 $9.95   ❑

The Business Traveler's Guide to Good Health on the Road edited by Karl Neumann, M.D., and Maury Rosenbaum. This innovative guide shows business travelers how to make smart food choices, exercise in planes, trains, automobiles, and hotel rooms, relieve stress, and more. Plus, this guide has a listing of hotels in the U.S. and Canada with fitness facilities. All this, presented with a generous seasoning of fun and interesting facts and tidbits, makes the book a must for every business traveler's expense list.

004233   ISBN 1-56561-036-9 $12.95 ❑

The Healthy Eater's Guide to Family & Chain Restaurants by Hope S. Warshaw, M.M.Sc., R.D. Here's the only guide that tells you how to eat healthier in over 100 of America's most popular family and chain restaurants. It offers complete and up-to-date nutrition information and suggests which items to choose and avoid.

004214   ISBN 1-56561-017-2 $9.95   ❑

Fat Is Not a Four-Letter Word by Charles Roy Schroeder, Ph.D. Through fascinating scientific, nutritional, and historical evidence, this controversial and insightful guide shows why millions of "overweight" people are unnecessarily knocking themselves out to look like fashion models. It offers a realistic approach to healthful dieting and exercise.

004095   ISBN 1-56561-000-8 $14.95   ❑

Exchanges for All Occasions by Marion Franz, R.D., M.S. Exchanges and meal planning suggestions for just about any occasion, sample meal plans, special tips for people with diabetes, and more.

004201   ISBN 1-56561-005-9 $12.95   ❑

Beyond Alfalfa Sprouts & Cheese: The Healthy Meatless Cookbook by Judy Gilliard and Joy Kirkpatrick, R.D., includes creative and savory meatless dishes using ingredients found in just about every grocery store. It also contains helpful cooking tips, complete nutrition information, and the latest exchange values.

004218   ISBN 1-56561-020-2 $12.95   ❑

One Year of Healthy, Hearty, & Simple One-Dish Meals by Pam Spaude and Jan Owan-McMenamin, R.D., is a collection of 365 easy-to-make healthy and tasty family favorites and unique creations that are meals in themselves. Most of the dishes take under 30 minutes to prepare.

004217   ISBN 1-56561-019-9 $12.95   ❑

Foods to Stay Vibrant, Young & Healthy by Audrey C. Wright, M.S., R.D., Sandra K. Nissenberg, M.S., R.D., and Betsy Manis, R.D. From tips on increasing bone strength to losing weight, here's everything women in midlife need to know to keep young and healthy through food. With authoritative advice from three of the country's leading registered dietitians, women over 40 can eat their way to good health and feel better than ever!

004256   ISBN 1-56561-057-1 $11.95   ❑

200 Kid-Tested Ways to Lower the Fat in Your Child's Favorite Foods by Elaine Moquette-Magee, M.P.H., R.D. For the first time ever, here's a much needed and asked for guide that gives easy, step-by-step instructions to cutting the fat in the most popular brand-name and home-made foods kids eat every day—without them even noticing.

004231   ISBN 1-56561-034-2 $12.95   ❑

Order by mail

Chronimed Publishing
P.O. Box 59032
Minneapolis, Minnesota 55459-9686

Place a check mark in the box next to the book(s) you would like sent. Enclosed is $_____. (Please add $3.00 to this order to cover postage and handling. Minnesota residents add 6.5% sales tax.)

Send check or money order, no cash or C.O.D.'s. Prices and availability are subject to change without notice.

Name _____

Address_____

City _____State _____Zip _____

Or
Order by phone: 1-800-848-2793
612-546-1146 (Minneapolis/St. Paul metro area).

■ Please have your credit card number ready.
■ Allow 4 to 6 weeks for delivery.
■ Quantity discounts available upon request.
■ Prices and availability subject to change without notice.